THE PRACTICE OF

Patient
Education

A Case Study Approach

THE PRACTICE OF
Patient Education
A Case Study Approach

Tenth Edition

Barbara Klug Redman RN, PhD, FAAN
Dean and Professor
Wayne State University College of Nursing
Detroit, Michigan

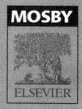

MOSBY

ELSEVIER

11830 Westline Industrial Drive
St. Louis, Missouri 63146

THE PRACTICE OF PATIENT EDUCATION: A CASE STUDY APPROACH

ISBN-13: 978-0-323-03905-5
ISBN-10: 0-323-03905-7

ISBN-13: 978-0-323-03905-5
ISBN-10: 0-323-03905-7

Executive Editor: Susan R. Epstein
Senior Developmental Editor: Maria Broeker
Publishing Services Manager: Deborah L. Vogel
Senior Project Manager: Steve Ramay
Designer: Amy Buxton

Printed in the United States of America

Last digit is the print number: 9 8 7 6 5 4 3 2 1

To the memories of Darlien and Harlan Klug.

Reviewers

Donell L. Campbell, RN, BA
Medical Surgical Manager
Providence Newberg Hospital
Newberg, Oregon

Esther H. Condon, PhD, RN
Professor of Nursing
Hampton University
Hampton, Virginia

Patricia J. Hutchison, RN, MSN, CDE
Education Coordinator
Grove City Medical Center
Grove City, Pennsylvania

Preface

This book is written for all health care providers who want to know more about how to teach patients and families. Because the book began as a nursing text and because nursing has such a rich philosophic and conceptual heritage in patient education, much of the background is still drawn from that field. Students should be ready to use the book when they recognize in their patients the need for learning, when they have enough knowledge to be able to teach the subject matter, and when they are competent in their interactions with patients.

The book is organized into two basic sections—the first describing the process of learning and teaching and the second reflecting major fields of patient education practice in place today. An entirely newly developed set of cases has been developed. Examples throughout the text are not meant to be exhaustive but are illustrative of the teaching-learning process.

This new edition features:
- Streamlined basics that can be used as the main text for a course or as a supplement to any clinically oriented course.
- Evidence-based patient education practice, with extensive citations to the research base.
- Multiple examples at every stage of the teaching process, which students can use as models to guide their own practice.
- Key issues in patient education such as literacy, use of patient decision aids, and multiple patient conditions for which organized patient education should be developed.
- Study questions with suggested answers.
- Multiple case examples for students to work to develop competency in managing real patient education problems.
- New strategies such as constructivist philosophy of learning in real settings, and motivational interviewing.
- Significant content in patient self-management of chronic conditions, the largest growing area of patient education.

Contents

Abbreviations Used

AEC	asthma education center
ADL	activities of daily living
AFDC	Aid to Families with Dependent Children
AMI	acute myocardial infarction
ANV	anticipatory nausea and vomiting
APN	advance practice nurse
ASMP	Asthma Self-Management Program
BGAT	blood glucose awareness training
BP	blood pressure; also DBP (diastolic blood pressure) and SBP (systolic blood pressure)
BSE	breast self-examination
BTS	Back to Sleep
CDC	Centers for Disease Control and Prevention
CDE	certified diabetes educator
CF	cystic fibrosis
CHF	congestive heart failure
CLS	child life specialist
COPD	chronic obstructive pulmonary disease
CPR	cardiopulmonary resuscitation
ED	emergency department
ESRD	end stage renal disease
HbA1C	glycolated hemoglobin
IBS	irritable bowel syndrome
JCAHO	Joint Commission for the Accreditation of Healthcare Organizations
LDL-C	low-density lipoprotein cholesterol; also HDL-C (high-density lipoprotein cholestero)
MCO	managed care organization
MDI	metered dose inhalers
MI	motivational interviewing
MRI	magnetic resonance imaging
MVP	mitral valve prolapse
NAEP	National Asthma Education and Prevention Program
NBAS	Brazelton Neonatal Behavioral Assessment Scale
NICU	neonatal intensive care unit
OA	osteoarthritis
OAS	Open Airways for Schools
PCA	patient controlled analgesia
PEF or PEFR	peak expiratory flow rate
PIL	patient information leaflet
PKU	phenylketonuria
PSA	prostate specific antigen
PTSD	posttraumatic stress disorder
RCT	randomized controlled trial
REALM	Rapid Estimate of Adult Literacy in Medicine
RT	respiratory therapist
SE	self-efficacy
SIDS	sudden infant death syndrome
SM	self-management
TOFHLA	Test of Functional Health Literacy in Adults
UK	United Kingdom
US	United States
WIC	Women, Infants, and Children

1

The Practice of Patient Education: Overview, Motivation, and Learning

Patient education is a central part of the practice of all health professionals. It is based on a set of theories, on research findings, and on skills that must be learned and practiced.

Patient education services are delivered during direct caregiving by health care practitioners and also in separate programs such as a diabetes self-management program. The legal base of patient education has been developed through case law and regulations governing professional practice and accreditation of health care institutions and most especially through the doctrine of informed consent. Its ethical base is still being defined. Ethical practice requires the competent practice of patient education by professionals, avoidance of the harms that this intervention can induce (such as debilitating confusion or loss of self-confidence), and serious examination of the reasons for asking the patient or family members to change beliefs and practices, frequently at great cost to themselves. It must be devoid of gender, ethnic, and age bias and effective for persons of widely varied levels of formal education.

THE PROCESS OF PATIENT EDUCATION

Patient education is practiced by a process of diagnosis and intervention. The needs-assessment phase determines the nature of a need and motivation to learn, and goals are mutually set with the patient. The intervention is constructed to provide instructional stimulation for the exact learning needs that patients have. Evaluation occurs throughout instruction, summarized at periodic intervals to determine whether the outcome goals are being met. Reteaching is frequently necessary because it is not possible to accurately predict which instructional intervention will yield the desired learning by a particular patient. In most instances, follow-up reinforcement and reteaching are needed over time, particularly for patients who are managing chronic health problems or learning how to prevent them.

The process of teaching can be summarized as follows:

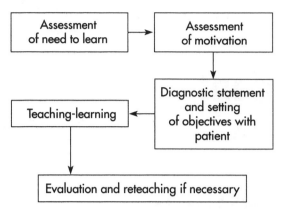

Little is known about how this process is actually used by practitioners, but what seems clearest is that it does not flow in an orderly, sequential fashion, as shown in the preceding diagram. One starts at the beginning of the process but subsequently skips from step to step; however, the elements do serve as checkpoints to ensure that the relevant variables that affect the teaching-learning activity have been considered. Although teaching does not have a complete set of commonly used diagnostic categories, the objectives can serve such a purpose. In addition, as nursing diagnostic categories have been refined and expanded, they have become useful but incomplete in categorizing patient learning needs.

The teaching process can be seen as parallel to the nursing process in that each has an assessment, diagnosis, goals, intervention, and evaluation phase (Table 1-1). Because learning about health is pertinent to nursing practice, some general screening questions should be part of the general nursing assessment; for example, what do patients know, how do they perceive their present problems, what skills do they possess and do they have the confidence to use them? If at any time during care the continuing assessment indicates a patient learning problem that teaching can alleviate, a more refined assessment of need and readiness is made and that problem is dealt with through the teaching process.

Common errors in practice include (1) omission of assessment of the patient's need to learn, so that no activity in patient education is initiated, and (2) omission of any given step, for example, omitting the assessment of readiness, the setting of goals, or the systematic evaluation, but not omitting the actual intervention. Of course, it is impossible not to have at least implicit goals when one teaches, but the goals may not be related to a particular patient's readiness and the instruction may not be constructed to meet those goals.

With adequate practice, providers can become proficient in thinking through the required steps

TABLE 1-1	**Relationship of Teaching Process to Nursing Process**			
Assessment	**Diagnosis**	**Goals**	**Intervention**	**Evaluation**
Nursing Process				
General screening questions to detect patient's need to learn	One of problem statements may be a need to learn or a nursing diagnosis	Learning goals are a subset of goals	Teaching intervention may be delivered with other intervention	Evaluating whether nursing care outcome was met
Teaching Process				
Refined assessment of need and readiness to learn	Learning diagnosis	Setting of learning goals	Teaching	Evaluating learning

of the teaching process. They can learn to stimulate readiness and become sensitive to expressions of it that may be part of an ordinary conversation with the patient and can learn to organize care to elicit measurements of readiness.

MOTIVATION

Motivation is a term that describes forces acting on or within an organism that initiate, direct, and maintain behavior. Motivation also explains differences in the intensity and direction of behavior. In the teaching-learning situation, motivation addresses the willingness of the learner to embrace learning. The term *readiness* describes evidence of motivation at a particular time. This chapter discusses theories of motivation in general, with specific application to health. It also describes assessment of motivation as part of the teaching-learning process and presents teaching practices that stimulate and develop motivation.

Six general theories of motivation can be used to direct learning in a variety of situations.[31]

Reinforcers. In behavioral learning theory the concept of motivation is tied closely to reinforcement of repeated behaviors. For example, behaviors that have been reinforced in the past are more likely to be repeated than are behaviors that have not been reinforced or that have been punished. Reinforcement histories and schedules of reinforcement help explain why some individuals learn better than others.

Needs. Satisfaction of needs for food, shelter, love, and maintenance of positive self-esteem explains the concept of motivation for other theorists. Persons differ in the degree of importance they attach to each of these needs. Satisfaction of three innate psychological needs for competence, autonomy, and relatedness enhance instrinsic (doing an activity for the inherent satisfaction) motivation and self-regulation. Excessive control and lack of connectedness disrupt motivation and thus sustained learning.[28]

Cognitive dissonance. Cognitive dissonance theory holds that individuals experience tension or discomfort when a deeply held value or belief is challenged by a psychologically inconsistent belief or behavior. To resolve the discomfort, patients may change a behavior or a belief, or they may develop justifications or excuses that resolve the inconsistency.

Attribution. To make sense of the world, individuals will often try to identify causes to explain why something has happened to them. Persons are particularly motivated to conduct attributional searches in ambiguous, extraordinary, unpredictable, or uncontrollable situations. Attributions may occur after a diagnosis, an exacerbation of chronic illness, an accidental injury, or the relief or cure of a symptom or illness. We know that attributions can have powerful effects on psychological adjustment, behavior, and morbidity. In a study of patients with myocardial infarctions, attributions of patients and their spouses (Why did this happen to me?) significantly predicted whether the family considered itself rehabilitated. Individuals make attributions about disease severity and treatment efficacy. They use these ideas to regulate self-management of their diseases.[16] Thus it is always important to know patients' beliefs about the cause of the current situation because their actions are guided by these attributions.

A concept central to attribution theory is *locus of control*. Those with an internal locus of control in a situation attribute success or failure to their own efforts or abilities. Those with an external locus of control believe that success or failure depends on luck, task difficulty, or other persons' actions.

Personality. Motivation in personality theory describes a general tendency to strive toward certain types of goals such as affiliation or achievement. An extreme motivation to avoid failure is learned helplessness, which causes persons to believe that they are doomed to failure no matter what. This behavior can arise from an inconsistent and unpredictable use of rewards and punishments by teachers. The problem can be avoided or alleviated by giving learners opportunities to realize success in small steps and by giving them immediate, positive feedback with consistent expectations and follow-through.

Coping styles may also be part of personality. Some individuals are vigilant and seek information from all available sources. If these persons find discrepancies in the information they receive, they feel anxious. Others use a coping style of avoidance. They want little information because it constitutes a source of stress. Monitors typically scan the environment for threat-relevant information and rehearse and amplify the threats cognitively, whereas blunters cope with aversive health events by distraction. Patients fare better psychologically, behaviorally, and physiologically when the information they receive is tailored to their coping style. Monitors do better when given more information that can be used constructively and more emotional support. Those with blunting styles do better with less information.[19]

Expectancy. Expectancy theories of motivation hold that a person's motivation to realize a goal depends on the perceived chance of success and on how much value that person places on success. The theory of reasoned action posits that volitional behavior is predicted by the person's intention to perform the behavior. Intention is, in turn, a function of beliefs about the consequences of the behavior and norms about the behavior that are held by significant others.[20]

Summaries of research have shown a powerful relationship between perceived self-efficacy (confidence that one can do the task) and adequate performance. How individuals judge their capabilities to produce and regulate events in their lives affects their motivation, their thought patterns, their behavior, and their emotions. Those who believe that they will not be able to cope well dwell on their personal deficiencies and imagine that potential difficulties will be more formidable than they really are. Self-efficacy increases notably when persons' experiences contradict their fears and when they gain new skills in managing threatening activities. Repeated failures lower self-efficacy, especially if failure occurs early in the course of events and does not reflect lack of effort or adverse external circumstances.[3,4]

Judgments about self-efficacy are based on the following sources of information: performance attainments (the most influential), vicarious experiences of observing the performance of others, verbal persuasion and other social influences,

and physiological states. Self-efficacy probes during a course of treatment can provide helpful guides for implementing a program of personal change. Adopting attainable subgoals that lead to more impressive future goals can provide the patient with clear markers of progress to verify a growing sense of self-efficacy.[3]

Finally, humanistic interpretations of motivation emphasize personal freedom, choice, self-determination, and a striving for personal growth. Although generally not expressed as a theory in the scientific sense, important assumptions made by humanists cause us to reflect on learners' resolutions to become motivated and to make their own decisions about whether to pursue a course of action.

Two theoretical models and an intervention to assess and stimulate motivation follow.

Health Belief Model

The health belief model[27] affirms that individuals are not likely to take a health action unless (1) they believe that they are susceptible to the ill health condition in question, (2) they believe that the condition would seriously affect their lives if they should contract it, (3) they believe that the benefits of action outweigh the barriers to action, and (4) they are confident that they can perform the action (self-efficacy). Cues such as an interpersonal crisis or the nature and severity of symptoms trigger action. This model, which is depicted in Figure 1-1, is an example of the value-expectancy approach, developed to explain an individual's health actions under conditions of uncertainty.

In patient education practice, the health belief model has been used to assess whether an individual holds these beliefs, and if not, to direct teaching at missing skills or information. Kloeblen and Batish[15] provide an example of the applicability of the health belief model to understand the intention among low-income pregnant women to permanently follow a high-folate diet for protection against neural tube defects. Items used to measure each construct in the model may be seen in Box 1-1. Among the group of women studied, perceived benefits were most predictive of intention to use folate.[15]

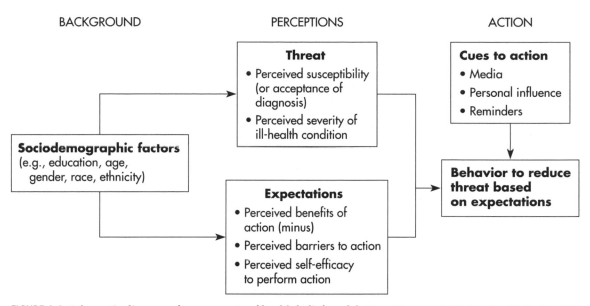

FIGURE 1-1 Schematic diagram of components of health belief model. (From Rosenstock IM, Strecher VJ, Becker MH: *The health belief model and HIV risk behavior change.* In Di Clemente RJ, Peterson JL, editors: *Preventing AIDS: theories and methods of behavioral interventions*, New York, 1994, Plenum Press.)

Transtheoretical Model

A second model relevant to motivation is the transtheoretical model of change. It holds that intentional change requires movement through discrete motivational stages over time, the active use of different processes of change at different stages, and modifications of cognitions, affect, and behaviors. Although it has been most thoroughly studied with addictive behaviors such as smoking, it is also useful for prediction of, and intervention in, behaviors more open to the effects of patient education, such as exercise, diet change, and management of chronic diseases such as diabetes and heart failure. Progression through the stages is not usually linear; for most health behavior problems the majority of individuals relapse and return to earlier stages of the model before eventually succeeding in maintaining change.

The stages of change are as follows[26]:

1. *Precontemplation.* Individuals are not considering change within the next 6 months. They may be resistant, have lack of knowledge, or be overwhelmed by the problem.

2. *Contemplation.* Individuals are seriously thinking about changing within the next 6 months, but, because of ambivalence, they may remain in this stage for years.

3. *Preparation.* Individuals are seriously planning to change within the next month and have already taken some steps toward action.

4. *Action.* This stage, which involves overt modification of the problem behavior, can last from 3 to 6 months.

5. *Maintenance.* This period begins after 6 months of continuous successful behavior change. Individuals can remain in maintenance from 3 to 5 years and still experience temptations to relapse.

In early stages the decisional balance is stronger for the cons—that is, against taking the action—than for the pros—that is, for taking it. Before action occurs, the balance must swing so that the pros outweigh the cons. For example, in the adoption of exercise behavior, the pros might include helping to relieve tension, liking the body better, having a more positive outlook on life, sleeping more soundly, and having more energy.

| **Box 1-1** | *Application of Health Belief Model for High Folate Diet* |

Perceived Susceptibility Statements

1. If I do not eat a diet high in folic acid before my pregnancy and very early in my pregnancy, I could have a baby with a neural tube defect (NTD), which is a type of birth defect.
2. I could get pregnant and my unborn baby could be sick without my even knowing it.
3. I could get pregnant sometime (besides now) and not know it right away.
4. I could have a baby with a birth defect someday.
5. I get colds and illnesses all of the time.

Perceived Severity Statements

1. Having an NTD, which is a type of birth defect, is a very serious condition.
2. Having an NTD would leave a child disabled for life.
3. Complications in an infant with an NTD are severe and could even result in death.
4. Having a baby with a birth defect would be very expensive.
5. Having a baby with a birth defect would negatively affect my social life, my family life, and my ability to work.

Perceived Benefits Statements

1. Eating more foods high in folic acid all of the time, even when I am not pregnant, could prevent or reduce my risk of having a baby with an NTD (a type of birth defect).
2. My family and friends would be proud of me if I improved my diet to contain more foods high in folic acid.
3. Improving my diet to include more foods high in folic acid could make me feel better and be a healthier person overall.
4. Changing my diet to include more foods high in folic acid all the time in case I get pregnant would make me feel good about myself.
5. Eating a diet high in folic acid all the time could save me money and time by helping to keep me from having a baby with an NTD, which would be expensive and would require a lot of time to care for.
6. Eating a diet high in folic acid all the time could help keep me healthy and help keep my baby healthy if I were to get pregnant again.

Perceived Barriers Statements

1. I think that eating a diet high in folic acid would be expensive.
2. I don't know enough about what foods are high in folic acid. I don't like most foods that are high in folic acid.
3. I think it would take too much time to change my diet to include more foods high in folic acid all of the time.
4. I think it would be too hard to change my diet to include more foods high in folic acid all of the time.
5. My friends and family would not like the changes in my diet if I tried to eat foods high in folic acid all of the time.

Self-Efficacy Statements

1. I am confident that I could eat a diet high in folic acid all of the time if I tried.
2. I feel that I would be able to follow a diet high in folic acid if I wanted to.

Cues to Action Statements

1. If a health professional reminded me to eat a diet high in folic acid when I came in for a doctor's visit, that would help me remember to eat more foods high in folic acid all of the time.
2. Seeing something on television about folic acid would help remind me to follow a diet high in folic acid all of the time.
3. If a friend or someone I know told me about folic acid, that would help me to be sure I get plenty of folic acid in my diet all of the time.
4. Reading pamphlets or seeing posters about folic acid would help me remember to eat more foods high in folic acid all of the time.
5. Have you ever talked about folic acid with someone else, such as a nutritionist, doctor, nurse, friend, or family member? (in % yes)
6. Do you know someone who had a baby with an NTD or who has lost a baby with an NTD? (in % yes)
7. Have you ever had a baby with a NTD? (in % yes)

From Kloeblen AS, Batish SS: Understanding the intention to permanently follow a high folate diet among a sample of low-income pregnant women according to the Health Belief Model. *Health Educ Res* 14:327-338, 1999.

The cons might include feeling too exhausted to exercise, exercise taking too much time, and feeling uncomfortable from getting out of breath.[25] Predictably, perceived self-efficacy (confidence that I can succeed in taking this action) is lowest during the early stages and rises as one progresses.

Typically, about 40% of populations at risk are in the precontemplation stage, another 40% are in the contemplation stage and stuck there for long periods of time by ambivalence, and only 10% to 20% are in the preparation stage. These ratios hold across a number of behaviors: smoking, alcohol and substance abuse, anxiety and panic disorders, eating disorders and obesity, high-fat diets, AIDS prevention, mammography screening, unplanned pregnancy prevention, and sedentary lifestyle. Patients with diabetes in the preparation and action stages achieved significantly larger reductions in hemoglobin A1c levels in a

shorter time than did patients in the combined precontemplation-contemplation stage.[24] Relapse occurs from action or maintenance to an earlier stage, although usually not as far back as precontemplation.[29] It is essential that the instructional strategy be matched to the stage; many educational programs are implicitly designed for individuals who are ready to take action. Box 1-2 provides examples of questions asked to determine what stage an individual is in and intervention approaches appropriate for the various stages for patients with heart failure.

Motivational Interviewing

Motivational interviewing (MI) is a client-centered, goal-directed counseling style originally developed to address substance abuse problems and later adapted to facilitate a broader spectrum of health behavior changes, such as adherence

---

| **Box 1-2** | *Questions about Stage of Change and Response Options for Persons with Heart Failure* |

Questions with Definitions

Do you exercise 3 times a week for at least 20 minutes each time?

Exercise includes brisk walking, riding a stationary bicycle, swimming, or other exercise of similar intensity advised for you. Activities that are primarily sedentary, such as bowling or playing golf with a cart, would not be considered exercise.

Do you drink 2 L (2 qt) or less of fluid a day (water, sodas, coffee, tea, juice)?

Have you eliminated high-sodium (salty) foods from your diet?

High-sodium foods include canned vegetables; processed foods such as deli meat, prepared gravy and sauces, frozen dinners; "fast food" (such as pizza, fried chicken, burgers, French fries), and snacks (such as potato chips, corn chips, salted nuts). Foods also become high in sodium when salt is added to them during cooking or at the table.

If Applicable:

Have you quit smoking cigarettes (or other tobacco products)?

Have you quit drinking alcohol (beer, wine, liquor)?

Have you been trying to lose weight by dieting (eating fewer foods, smaller portions, or less fattening foods)?

Response Options

Maintenance:	Yes, I have been for more than 6 months.
Action:	Yes, I have been for less than 6 months.
Preparation:	No, but I am planning to start in the next 30 days.
Contemplation:	No, but I am planning to start in the next 6 months.
Precontemplation:	No, and I don't plan to start in the next 6 months.

From Paul S and Sneed NV: Strategies for behavior change in patients with heart failure, *Am J Crit Care* 13:305-313, 2004. Used by permission of Oxford University Press.

to antiretroviral therapy among persons with HIV and contraceptives and helping at-risk prediabetic clients develop therapeutic lifestyle changes to reduce the diabetes risk. It provides a way of working with patients who may not seem ready to make the behavioral change considered necessary by the health practitioner. MI follows five counseling techniques aimed at helping clients resolve ambivalence about a health behavior: (1) expressing empathy, (2) developing discrepancy, (3) avoiding argument, (4) rolling with resistance, and (5) supporting self-efficacy.[1]

The patient does most of the talking, articulates and resolves her own ambivalence. The practitioner recognizes patient ambivalence and creates and amplifies any discrepancy between the patient's current behavior and her goals so that the patient presents the argument for change. Argumentation or direct persuasion is considered counterproductive and likely to produce defensiveness or resistance. The patient is encouraged to think about her current satisfaction with life and what the future looks like, both if she continues as she is and if she changes her behavior. The techniques of MI function to arouse cognitive dissonance in the patient by focusing on ambivalence and inconsistencies and then controlling the direction chosen for dissonance reduction, resolved by focusing on the patient's wants, expectations, beliefs, fears, and hopes and on the inconsistencies between these and the problematic behavior. Few controlled trials evaluate the efficacy of MI with health problems.[7]

Tables 1-2 through 1-4 provide examples of MI stages in at-risk prediabetic patients who should adopt a healthy diet, decrease weight, and increase exercise to prevent or delay onset of type 2 diabetes. Up to 7% weight loss and 150 minutes of physical activity per week are more effective in preventing diabetes than is standard pharmacologic therapy. Note the strategies the provider uses to move the patient (AJ) through the stages of motivation for change.[9]

LEARNING

Instructional practices are also based on the psychology of learning and on material that has produced results for practitioners in the past. Although bright, motivated individuals can learn a great deal without a teacher, their efforts to learn can be quite inefficient. Individuals who need to learn health information and skills, even if they are motivated, often do not have sufficient orientation to health matters to attain the goal alone. Learning is defined as change in an individual caused by experience and does not include changes caused by development.[31]

Theories of Learning

Learning involves changing to a new state—it is a state that persists. What can be learned? New thinking strategies, new motor skills, new attitudes, and new confidence are learned in complex patterns that can promote and sustain a new performance. General conditions exist (such as reinforcement and transfer) that are applicable to all kinds of learning and learners. Particular conditions that facilitate particular kinds of learning are also present.

Current learning theories may be classified into two broad categories: behavioral and cognitive, with Bandura's social cognitive theory containing many key elements of both.[4] Recently, theories/philosophies of constructivism suggest that learners are helped to construct their own meaning in real environments—frequently in teams working together to solve problems. Conscious learning and conceptualization emerge from this activity instead of preceding it, transmitted by teacher to learner in artificial environments.[14]

Behavioral Learning Theory

The most important principle of behavioral learning theory is that behavior changes according to its immediate consequences. Pleasurable consequences strengthen behavior (reinforce it), whereas unpleasant consequences weaken it. Reinforcers may be food, water, warmth, praise, recognition, grades, or paychecks, varying from one individual to another. Extinction is a process used to decrease a previously reinforced behavior by ceasing reinforcement. Also, punishment delivered immediately in response to a particular behavior may decrease that behavior; however, the results of punishment are unpredictable.

TABLE 1-2	**Establishing Rapport and Building Motivation for Change**
Interaction	**Strategy/Behavior**
Nurse: [AJ], we have about 45 minutes to talk today and, from what I understand, you are here about some concerns with your diabetic test results. Tell me more about what concerns you have.	Developing rapport Open-ended question
AJ: Well, I don't know. My doctor wanted me to see you. He told me I need to lose weight and start exercising. I've always been a little heavy, I eat what I want, and I don't exercise. However, I've generally always been in pretty good health. My mother and father died of complications of diabetes. My mother died of kidney failure, and my dad had multiple amputations. Genetically, the doctor probably thinks I'll get diabetes one day like them. Do we have to talk about this?	Ambivalence Negating
Nurse: We can talk about anything you want to. You mentioned diabetic complications, family history, losing weight, and exercise. That's a lot of items, but this time is yours. What concerns you the most?	Rolling with resistance Simple reflection Open-ended question
AJ: Well, he keeps telling me I need to exercise and lose weight.	
Nurse: Tell me how you feel about your current weight and physical activity.	Open-ended statement
AJ: I don't really think I'm fat. As far as exercise, I do enough at work. I work in a restaurant. I'm on my feet all day.	Ambivalence
Nurse: It's good to hear you have a positive self-image. How do you think weight and exercise are linked with diabetes?	Affirmation Open-ended question
AJ: When my parents had high sugars, losing weight and exercising seemed to help bring the sugar levels down a bit.	
Nurse: You're right, eating right and exercising help your body become more sensitive to insulin. This allows your body to use insulin better, whereas in diabetes, you are not able to use insulin effectively (pancreas secretes insulin). Insulin lowers your sugar levels. You had a glucose tolerance test to check your sugar levels, and the test came back abnormally high.	Information giving Summarizing
AJ: Yeah, something like that. What does the high number mean? I don't have diabetes, do I?	Information seeking Information giving
Nurse: No, not yet. I have the result and the level was 190 mg/dL. The normal value is ≥140 mg/dL but < 200 mg/dL so 190 mg/dL is high. You have impaired glucose tolerance. This is the stage right before you actually get diabetes. It can lead to type 2 diabetes, where the pancreas does not secrete enough insulin or the body cells are resistant to what insulin is supposed to do, which is to lower your blood sugar. If your sugar level remains within those high levels over time, it can cause a series of events in your body that can lead to diabetes and its complications, like what your parents had, and probably even to heart disease.	Moving away from MI
Alternative response: You are concerned about getting diabetes?	Reflective listening Reflection
AJ: Well, I don't want diabetes.	Beginning of change talk

Reproduced with permission from Carino JL, Coke L, Gulanik M: Using motivational interviewing to reduce diabetes risk. *Prog Cardiovasc Nursing* 12:149-154, 2004. Copyright 2004 by CHF, Inc.

TABLE 1-3	Eliciting Change Talk
Interaction	**Strategy/Behavior**
Nurse: Your risk level is higher for diabetes because of your elevated sugar levels, your family history, being overweight, and not exercising. Changing your diet and losing some weight are things you can do to reduce your risk. AJ: That's too many things you're telling me. I can't change who I am, especially my heredity.	Redirecting the conversation
Nurse: You are right. You can't change the things that physically make up who you are, but there are some things you can do to lower the risk of getting diabetes. What do you think you can change? AJ: I guess I can eat less or watch closer what I eat since I eat so much junk. I probably need to exercise, too. Does doing all these things mean I won't get diabetes?	Affirming Evocative question Brainstorming
Nurse: There are no guarantees, but we know that changing diet and exercising more does help. On a scale of 0-10 with 0 being not important and 10 being most important, how would you rate the importance of doing something about your diabetes risk? AJ: Eight	Assessing importance
Nurse: That's pretty high. Then making a change is important to you? AJ: Yes, if it means I won't get diabetes.	Affirming
Nurse: On the same scale, how would you rate your confidence for making a health change to reduce your risk? AJ: Five, because I love to eat. I've failed a diet before, and I'm not very athletic.	Assessing confidence
Nurse: What needs to happen in order to move it to an 8? AJ: I think I would feel more confident if I had a partner doing this with me, or if I knew I can do this on a consistent basis.	Elaborating
Nurse: What would be the advantages and disadvantages of doing something about your risk? AJ: Well, I may not get diabetes for one thing. I would be healthier, feel more energized, look better, and I would feel better about myself. On the other hand, I may need to spend time and money on losing weight and exercising.	Exploring decisional balance Looking forward
Nurse: Tell me more about the second part—about time and money regarding weight and exercise. *Alternative Response: [Focus on the positive part of the statement.] So, doing something about your risk factors would make you feel better and reduce your chance of getting diabetes?* AJ: I might have to spend money to buy special foods, buy exercise clothes, or pay to join a health club. Then again, if I can do it, it's probably worth doing all this than paying to get my kidneys washed out.	Elaborating Change talk
Nurse: What would be the worst thing to you if you did nothing right now? AJ: I guess I'd continue to gain weight, be unhealthy, and wind up getting diabetes and maybe eventually end up like my parents.	Querying extremes

TABLE 1-3 Eliciting Change Talk—cont'd	
Interaction	**Strategy/Behavior**
Nurse: Have there been any other behavior changes you have tried where you were successful?	Looking back
AJ: Yeah, I quit smoking. That was the hardest thing I ever had to do! It took me 2 years to really quit smoking, and that was hard.	
Nurse: Wow! I really admire your will power and success. Knowing you have successfully quit smoking, how might you use that experience to successfully plan to shed a few pounds and do some walking?	Affirming Elaborating Exploring goals/values
Alternative Response: [Focus on one behavior change at a time. The client is more motivated to modify diet than exercise.]	
AJ: Well, I really like being social. I can get my daughter to join me since she is very overweight and want to lose a few pounds. I can get some coworkers to do Weight Watchers,* and we can all count points together. Some coworkers and I can go walking during our lunch break. Even better, since I love shopping, I can walk around the nearby mall.	Brainstorming Change talk
Nurse: I see you have lots of creative ideas. Tell me a little bit about the part about getting your daughter to join you.	Affirming Elaborating
AJ: Well, my daughter is only 15, and the doctor said she's 50 pounds overweight. I want her to be healthy, but she follows my example. I figure if I do things differently, she may follow.	
Nurse: So you really value being a healthy person, but you don't see yourself doing healthy actions for yourself or your daughter?	Exploring goals/values Creating discrepancy
AJ: No, I guess not when I think about the junk I eat.	
Nurse: Sounds like you are not happy with all these things because it makes you feel unhealthy.	Reflection
AJ: Yeah, but I don't think I'm that fat. I do try and eat better.	Resistance
Nurse: It seems that even if you feel a little overweight, you still feel good about yourself in many ways.	Reframing
AJ: Yeah, but there's no way I'm going to lose the weight to look like a supermodel.	Resistance
Nurse: No one is asking you to look like a supermodel. Losing weight means decreasing your risk and being healthier.	Coming along side
AJ: I do want to be healthier so I don't get diabetes.	Envisioning

*Weight Watchers International, Inc. (New York, NY).

Reproduced with permission from Carino JL, Coke L, Gulanik M: Using motivational interviewing to reduce diabetes risk. *Prog Cardiovasc Nursing* 12:149-154, 2004. Copyright 2004 by CHF, Inc.

The Premack principle theorizes that a particular behavior performed by a person frequently can be used to reinforce a low-frequency behavior. Shaping involves applying reinforcements in accordance with gradually changing criteria. As the performer begins to roughly approximate the target behavior, closer approximations of the final response are needed before reinforcement can be delivered.[31,35]

In teaching, one must be sure that effective reinforcement is applied to a well-defined behavior so that learners will understand what they

TABLE 1-4 Commitment to Change	
Interaction	**Strategy/Behavior**
Nurse: What are some things you think you can do?	Shifting focus
AJ: I guess I can try walking a day or two during the week.	Open-ended question
Nurse: If your risk for getting diabetes is clear to you and you had to do this, could you do it?	Change talk Supporting self-efficacy
AJ: I suppose I could…	Change talk
Nurse: We have about 10 minutes left, why don't we come up with a plan for walking?	Developing plan and goals
AJ: Yeah, I can only concentrate on one thing at a time. Let me get past this exercise thing first. It sounds easier. I can walk. I walk at work a lot.	Change talk
Nurse: I want you to know, though, that it's brisk walking that counts.	
AJ: Well, 15 minutes of walking a day doesn't sound too bad, I can walk during my lunch break or something. Then I can work my way up to more walking later.	Brainstorming Change talk
Nurse: That sounds great!	Affirmation

Reproduced with permission from Carino JL, Coke L, Gulanik M: Using motivational interviewing to reduce diabetes risk. *Prog Cardiovasc Nursing* 12:149-154, 2004. Copyright 2004 by CHF, Inc.

did to warrant the reward. As new behaviors are learned, reinforcement is frequent; however, after behaviors are established, reinforcement is given at random to encourage persistence of the behavior.

Staffs in nursing homes use these principles to teach shaving and dressing behavior to residents, reinforcing each step of the process and building to the entire behavior.

Cognitive Learning Theory

In cognitive theory, learning is the development of insights or understandings that provide a potential guide for behavior. New insights lead to a reorganization of the individual's cognitive structure, which is stored internally in visual images and in propositional networks and schemata to organize information. Within this framework, learning makes change in behavior possible, although not necessary. Motivation to take action results from a need to make sense of the world and solve problems. In contrast to behavioral theories that focus on the new behavior to be learned, the cognitive view emphasizes understanding of concepts and theories in the subject matter and general skills and abilities such as reasoning and problem solving.[35]

Teachers using this theory determine the schemata of the learner and organize content so that it can be assimilated easily into the existing schema. Some learning can be described as an accumulation of new information in memory; however, the basic goal is to direct a longitudinal development of increasingly sophisticated mental models. Each level of learning addresses a larger set of problems. Novices can relate only superficially to the problem area or to the subject matter and must use pre-existing schemata to interpret these isolated pieces of data. Experts, on the other hand, quickly identify the problem and know how to approach it, consolidate information in meaningful ways, and monitor and accurately predict the outcome of their performance.[11] In contrast to general learning skills, expertise is increasingly viewed as specific to a particular domain of knowledge or thought.

Social Cognitive Theory

Social cognitive theory as developed by Bandura[4] is largely a cognitive theory, but incorporates principles of behaviorism. According to this theory, humans respond primarily to cognitive representations of the environment rather than to the environment itself.

Individuals acquire information, values, attitudes, moral judgments, standards of behavior, and new behaviors through observing others. Infants who are several months old model behavior with competence and continue to do so throughout their lives. Individuals can learn and formulate rules of behavior by observing persons, films or videotapes of models, symbolic models (written accounts of a performance), or sets of instructions (compressed accounts of a performance). This coded information serves as a guide for future action. The learner also gets information about the probable consequences of modeled action. Individuals visualize themselves executing the correct sequence of actions; therefore, cognitive rehearsals and actual performances increase the proficiency of individuals, give them a sense of efficacy, and reduce the tendency to forget learned behaviors.

In social cognitive theory, behavior is regulated by expectations for similar outcomes on future occasions. Individuals will persist for some time in actions that go unrewarded on the expectation that their efforts will eventually produce rewarding results. Extrinsic incentives are especially necessary in early stages of developing competencies (such as playing the piano) until competence becomes self-rewarding. The natural social environment is often inconsistent, contradictory, and inattentive. To ensure that the individual's newly acquired skills generalize and endure under these less than favorable circumstances, transitional practices must gradually approximate those of the natural social environment.

Much behavior is motivated and regulated by internal standards and self-evaluative reactions to the individual's own actions, including self-incentives and self-concepts of efficacy. To function competently requires skills and perceived self-efficacy. Perceived self-efficacy is a belief in one's ability to realize a certain level of performance. It must be distinguished from outcome efficacy, which judges the likely consequence certain such behaviors will produce. Judgments of self-efficacy are based on four principal sources of information: (1) performance attainments, the strongest of the sources, which involve acting out the desired behavior, with repeated failures lowering self-efficacy; (2) vicarious experiences through observing the performances of others, especially if the model is similar to the learner in ability, age, sex, and experiences; (3) verbal persuasion; and (4) perceived physiological states from which individuals partly judge their capability, strength, and vulnerability. Self-efficacy also lessens unsettling emotions such as stress and depression.[4,5] For example, cardiac rehabilitation programs are structured to provide information from these four sources, and the patient's perceived self-efficacy to perform various tasks is closely related to whether he or she will attempt those activities.

Types of Learning

Transfer of Learning

Transfer of learning, the effect of prior learning on subsequent learning, is one of the most important products of education, inasmuch as no learner can practice for all situations that will arise. It is more efficient for an individual to learn general information, skills, and ways of thinking and apply them to a variety of situations than to learn specifically for each situation. Teaching for transfer is based on evidence that individuals forget nonsense material and isolated facts. However, individuals remember general ideas, attitudes, ways of thinking, and skills that are meaningful to them and that they have thoroughly learned and applied.

For the transfer of learning to occur, individuals must also recognize that the new situation is similar to previously learned situations and they must remember which specific thoughts or behaviors are appropriate. In behavioral learning theory, transfer has an increased probability for responses occurring in the future because of past performance or because of the appearance of identical stimuli. In cognitive learning theory, transfer is not automatic; when it occurs, it is in the form of generalizations, concepts, or insights that have been developed in one situation and are being used in other situations.

Many studies provide evidence that generally positive transfer increases when overall training and application conditions coincide. Practice in a variety of contexts enhances transfer (less like the original learning). Indeed, extensive, varied practice based on imitating a model and driven by reinforcers can lead to the automatic triggering of a well-learned behavior in a new context. Use of examples aids transfer, especially if one extracts the rule from the current example and uses it in new situations.[29] Instruction must be planned to ensure that transfer will occur and must continue until the individual has mastered the learning. Experience shows that some patients need repeated education to master initial skills[2] and certainly intermittently over the course of a chronic disease.

Memory

Forgetting learned material is one of the banes of our existence. Not using learned material, interference of other learning, loss during reorganization of ideas, and motivated forgetting (which may be subconscious) constitute explanations for not remembering learned materials. Nevertheless, ideas are remembered for a long time, whereas facts are not.

The cognitive process involves the following: (1) selective perception of stimuli from the environment; (2) storage in short-term memory persisting for as long as 20 seconds; (3) encoding (leaves short-term memory and enters long-term memory); (4) storage in a meaningful mode as concepts, propositions, schema, and imagery in long-term memory; (5) retrieval; (6) response generation; (7) performance (patterns of activity that can be observed); and (8) feedback. Instruction can aid each of these steps by providing, for example, differentiation of features facilitating selective perception, verbal instruction or pictures that suggest encoding schemes, or cues that aid

retrieval. Retrieval time is slow except for the short-term memory, which holds only six to nine items. Forgetting is characteristically a progressive loss of precise information about an event rather than the total loss of a stored item and usually occurs because of the ineffectiveness of search and retrieval processes, sometimes precipitated by fear or overload.

Information is stored in long-term memory in networks of connected facts or concepts called schemata. Information that fits into an existing schema is more easily understood, learned, and retained than is information that does not.[31]

Ways to increase memory retention include fostering intent to learn and to remember, overlearning, finding meaning in material to be learned, applying newly learned material to practical situations (practicing), rehearsing remembering, chunking information (related ideas together) to decrease memory load, using organizing strategies and visual imagery, learning over a period of time, and teaching to the learner's learning style. Use of projects or plays gives learners vivid images they can remember.

Ley[17] completed a series of studies on patient memory of clinical advice, which is summarized in an excellent article. Neither age nor intelligence showed any consistent relationship with recall. Diagnostic statements were best recalled and those concerned with instructions and advice most poorly recalled. These findings seemed to result from perceived "importance" effects. Four methods were found to increase recall: use of shorter words and sentences, explicit categorization, repetition, and use of concrete-specific rather than general-abstract statements (general: "You must lose weight"; specific: "You must lose 7 pounds"). Use of these tactics plus giving instructions and advice and stressing their importance resulted in significant differences in the amount of information recalled by patients.

Professionals have been shocked and dismayed at patient recall of informed consent conversations that generally include explanation of diagnosis, the nature of the illness, proposed surgery, risk of death or complications, benefits, and alternate methods of management, with the chances for failure or success. Patients frequently remember fewer than half the items covered, as verified against recordings of the initial conversation. Certainly, use of the approaches just outlined would improve retention.

Problem Solving

Problem solving is frequently a desired goal in learning situations. Problem tasks are more complex if they have one or more of the following characteristics: (1) incompletely defined alternatives, (2) existence of a number of subproblems, (3) several ways to reach the goal, (4) need for a large number of information sources to solve the problem, or (5) a rapidly changing problem situation.[8] Problem solving can be broken into a series of steps: (1) identification of the problem, (2) determination of possible actions and their probable results, (3) selection of one action, (4) implementation of the chosen action, and (5) evaluation of problem-solving effectiveness. Frequently, breaking the problem into parts is helpful. Learners may need help at any of the stages of problem solving. Assessing this need can be accomplished by problem solving out loud or by teaching a novice learner how to solve the problem.

Families that cope with advanced cancer vary significantly in their abilities to think through cancer-related problems and to carry out actions to minimize these problems. Problem-solving education is a relatively new approach, designed to bolster the ability of families to help themselves. In one program[8] patients and families were taught problem-solving skills, supplemented by a home care guide that used this approach and that involved active practice working through hypothetical problems and the family's own problems. Although this study did not have a control group, before and after measures showed better problem-solving skills and confidence post intervention.[2]

Attitude Learning and the Effect of Mood

Attitudes pervade all spheres of learning. They may be defined as learned, emotionally toned predispositions to react in particular ways toward an object, an idea, or a person. Values, which are similar but more permanent, are expressions of how individuals believe an object or relationship affects them. Over the years feelings are developed, become well established, and are reflected in behavior. Often we do not realize that we are acquiring attitudes. Membership in groups, particularly primary ones, seems to influence acquisition of attitudes.

Suggestions for teaching attitudes follow directly from knowledge about how they are learned and include using someone to teach whose attitudes the learner can view and imitate. This model might not be a health care professional but possibly another patient with whom the learner can identify, which is the reason for establishing colostomy and ileostomy clubs and other such groups. Another way of influencing attitudes is to provide satisfying experiences so that the person develops a positive response to ideas or feelings associated with the experiences. For example, personnel in a health care clinic should try to provide experiences of the sort that help patients have positive feelings about the clinic.

Mood, especially depression, is commonly understood to interfere with learning. For example, after an inpatient diabetes education program, some patients failed to show improvement in glycemic control during the first 3 months. Investigation showed that these patients were depressed, underscoring the importance of screening and treating depression in persons with diabetes.[2] Depressive disorders are found among others with heart disease, stroke, and end-stage renal disease with prevalence rates reaching as high as 40%. Highly negative beliefs about their illness (which may not correlate with objective measures of disease severity) may contribute to depression[12]; correcting these could be helpful.

Psychomotor Learning

Anyone recalling the awkwardness of a puppy or a child, or the unsteadiness of an old man, and comparing it with the sure coordination of a skilled artist can observe a variation in motor skills. These skills can vary with strength, reaction time, speed, balance, precision, and flexibility of tissues. Motor skills are usually composed of an ordered sequence of movement that must be learned. Separate parts of a motor act can be learned and practiced separately as part-skills.

To execute a particular skill, a person must possess a neuromuscular system that is capable of performing the skill and must have an ability to form a mental image of the act. A mental image is created when the learner watches a demonstration that shows the skill and points out relevant cues for a successful performance. Relevant cues often involve muscular cues of balance and pull; cues may also be seen or heard. When learning to walk with crutches, a person must see the floor or objects that might get in the way, hear persons approach from behind, and feel whether he or she is balanced. The cues must be obvious to the beginner and often are not noticed much in advance of the action. The person experienced in using the motor skill can use many cues rather than just the obvious ones. He or she is not confused by irrelevant cues, attending to them with less conscious concentration. Also, the person experienced in certain motor skills reacts faster and can take advantage of cues far in advance of action. The goal is a smooth, coordinated sequence of action with a minimum expenditure of energy.

The learner practices to develop a proficient performance. The mental image is a guide. At first, however, the teacher may need to guide the person's body so that he or she experiences the physical sensations that accompany correct motions. For example, one might guide a child's hands as she learns to drink from a cup. It is best for the learner to practice in a situation that provides cues similar to those in the environment where the skill will be used. For example, the person with a colostomy is taught in a setting that simulates a bathroom at home. During the crucial early stages of practice, information about the patient's progress, or lack of it, is important. Learners often need help in judging their own performances, even though they can judge someone else's. Eventually, learners receive messages from their own physical sensations and can decide whether their objectives have been accomplished.

It is generally recommended that practice periods be short and infrequent enough to avoid fatigue. If intervals between practices are too long, the learner may forget. Once a motor skill has been learned, it can be quickly recaptured even after an interval of many years.

Cognitive Learning

Cognitive learning theory holds that behavior and mood[12] is structured by the way people think about their experiences. Research on the structure of lay theories of health consistently finds five dimensions around which the experience of illness is organized: identity, cause, consequences, time line, and controllability. An individual's representation of a particular illness is made up of his or her answers to these questions. In Western society, having a causal theory about one's illness is related to better adjustment.[30] These schemas are important to know. For example, representations of medication show that patients interpret side effects as a sign that the drug is working and absence of them as distressing. Adherence issues may be explained by beliefs that if medicine is taken continuously it becomes less effective and carries the risk of dependence or addiction and that it is important to give the body a rest. Research shows that medication representations correlate with adherence.[13]

Concept mapping provides an opportunity to understand an individual patient's cognitive representations in an area in which learning is important to tailoring the content of instruction. This technique involves identifying key concepts in a subject matter and their linkages, thus describing the individual mental model. The mental model or cognitive map of a woman living with lupus may be found in Figure 1-2.

Current learning theory stresses use of authentic (real world) whole learning tasks, not hypothetical ones or tasks broken into small subskills. Yet, the complexity of real situations can hamper learning because there are so many things to remember and they all relate to each other, described as more or less cognitive load. Providing novice learners with worked examples

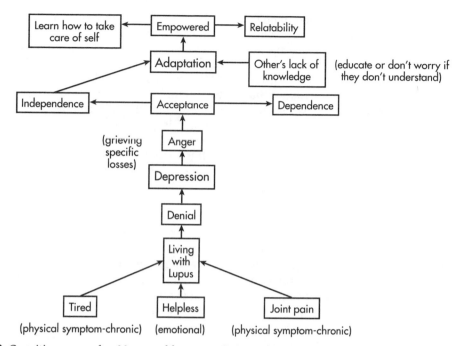

FIGURE 1-2 Cognitive map of a 33-year-old woman living with lupus. Note: Statements in parentheses are additional explanations by the participant. (From Wiginton KL: Illness representations: mapping the experience of lupus. *Health Educ Behav* 26:443-453, 1999.)

is helpful, as is sequencing learning from simple to complex over time and providing initial schemas to which learners can add.[33]

Cultural Differences in Learning

Although individuals within cultures differ widely, using group traditions in learning styles will usually yield more efficient and effective learning. Poor persons and ethnic minorities frequently rely on the oral tradition. Benavides-Vaello and others[6] describe working with such a population in south Texas with a high incidence of diabetes. They used focus groups (oral) to gather information on differences between groups in which diabetes was well controlled and those in which it was not. A high level of knowledge and confidence (self-efficacy) in their ability to manage their diabetes and take control of their health was found among those with well-controlled diabetes, and among others self-management skills appeared

to be disorganized with varying motivation and lack of self-confidence. Those in the latter group had difficulty articulating what they needed to know and how they could best learn. Culturally appropriate instructional videos, provision of blood glucose monitors and supplies, appropriate incorporation of home remedies, and teaching by others from their cultural group whose success they could model were key.

Developmental Phases

Adult Learning

The dominant current theory of adult learning builds on the cognitive tradition; the kind of learning most characteristic of the adult phase is transformative learning. The challenges of adulthood involve a process of traveling through an uncertain number of changes that transform the individual. A disorienting dilemma or an integrative circumstance usually provides motivation to reflect about one's perspectives and assumptions and to conclude that previous approaches are no longer adequate. Although adult learners do not return to old perspectives once transformation occurs, passages involve difficult negotiation and compromise, stalling, and backsliding. Self-deception and failure are common. The crucial difference between this transformation lag and primary (child) socialization is that adults are capable of being critically reflective and children are not. Assistance with perspective change involves helping adults see their problems and providing access to alternate-meaning perspectives to help individuals interpret the unreality. Adult learners can then examine their assumptions critically by using stories and pictures that pose hypothetical dilemmas, with conflicting rules and assumptions in the areas of critical concern. Little is known about why some dilemmas lead to perspective transformation and others do not.[32]

Indeed, support groups often involve adults who come together in response to the same life dilemma. These groups foster critical reflection. They help the participants gain and apply insights to their own lives. One can study the outcomes of this kind of education by interviewing group participants and by comparing movement in problem awareness, expectations, and goals.[18] Health-threatening situations frequently cause individuals to feel disoriented and can precipitate self-reflection.

Adaptation to the usual auditory and memory changes that frequently accompany aging must be built into instruction. Learning through alternate modalities (e.g., use of audiotapes if one does not see well) is important. Decline in memory can be compensated for by providing short instructional sessions focused on a few skills. Frequent practice until the material is overlearned and use of memory aids such as pill boxes that organize doses of medication are helpful.

Learning in Children

Ability to learn depends on maturation, and a great deal of maturation occurs in childhood. Readiness to learn in childhood changes consid-erably, beginning with visual, auditory, and motion stimulation of infants. The primary dimension of children's development is the degree of differentiation they make between the self and others. Children move toward a clearer distinction between the internal and the external self. The general principles and comments about learning outlined in previous sections of this chapter are applicable to children within their readiness level.

Intellectual development moves from concrete to abstract. During the preschool years, children can use language to represent objects or experiences and can solve problems by direct manipulation of physical objects. Young children are egocentric and interested in only what affects them. They want explanations for everything but are not concerned with supplying reasons for their questions. If children have a background of direct nonverbal experience during the elementary school years, they can verbally manipulate relationships between ideas without having the objects present. As they grow toward adolescence and then adulthood, they gradually come to understand and manipulate relationships between abstractions without any reference to the concrete. Eventually, they can formulate and test hypotheses on the basis of the possible combinations of several ideas.

Children must develop motor skills and feelings, as well as grow intellectually. Developing trust in the first 2 years is crucial. At that point children become more autonomous—learning to walk, run, jump, and feed themselves. Between the ages of $3^1/_2$ and 7, children develop imagination and learn to take initiative. During the early school years they become industrious, turning their attention to the outside world. As adolescents they develop their identities.

Knowledge of growth and development suggests that teachers should determine realistic objectives and explain them in a way that children can understand. Allowing children to handle equipment, such as a breathing mask, seems to encourage acceptance of treatment. This is especially true during the years when direct nonverbal experience is important. Because children younger than 5 years experience egocentricity and fear of injury, they need to know how procedures will affect them. For example, it can be explained to children that during a chest x-ray examination they will just have to stand still, hold their breath for a few seconds, and not worry, because they will not feel anything.

Research has consistently reported limited periods of behavioral upset followed by rapid recovery after discharge from the hospital. (Children between 6 months and 4 years are the most vulnerable.) Young children, in particular, consider illness to be self-caused and punitive. It has been suggested that if a child is younger than 4 years, explanation of anatomy and physiology is not useful because the child does not have the necessary understanding and is prone to develop undesirable fantasies. There is confusion between cause and effect and lack of differentiation between illnesses. Separation anxiety in this age group is a primary problem. Therefore, teaching should stress that whenever possible the same provider needs to care for the child, and the parents should be encouraged to participate.

For children older than 7 years, more sophisticated language and drawings can be used. Children of school age also benefit from tours of hospital playrooms and wards and from discussion in which they can learn about their illness, its origins, and proposed plans of treatment. Because school-age children have a maturer concept of causality than younger children possess, they have the capacity to understand that neither illness nor treatment is imposed on them because of their own misdeeds. These children are able to cooperate with treatment because they can think before they act. Because they can express their feelings in words and have a greater grasp of time sequences, they can better tolerate a separation from their parents.

Children's health attitudes and behaviors show a critical period of change around the time they enter the third grade. Third graders are able to decide whether to report illness or injury. They have developed cognitive abilities, and they have learned the social rules that govern illness and when to seek care. By the sixth grade these abilities are refined.

Adolescents must master the ability to think in abstractions and to imagine the possibilities that are inherent in a variety of situations. Many adolescents need help in thinking through behavioral alternatives. They may need guidance through steps of problem solving and planning. Role playing in peer groups can help illustrate appropriate norms of behavior. It can also translate abstract information into stories that are easier to remember.

Chronically ill children become increasingly able to understand their illnesses as they develop intellectually. Cognitive development brings with it the ability to grasp the meaning of a poor prognosis or of functional limitations.

Adolescents frequently display particular thought patterns involving an imaginary audience or a personal fable, consistent with a stage of intense preoccupation with themselves. They believe that if everyone is watching them and thinking about them, thanks to the imaginary audience, they must be something special, unique, or different. Teenagers with chronic illness may stop taking medications because they believe they are special and different and can manage without the medications. Believing that they are immune to the natural laws that other persons must obey can also cause them not to use contraceptives. Unprotected intercourse may not be viewed as a risk by the adolescent.[10] Pestrak and Martin[23] believe that many adolescents are functioning at a cognitive level that renders them unable to practice most forms of birth control effectively. The authors conclude that the effective practice of birth control requires that individuals accept their sexuality and acknowledge that they are sexually active, anticipate the present, and view potential future sexual encounters realistically.

Pridham, Adelson, and Hansen[25] have developed a useful tool (Table 1-5) describing how features of development are pertinent in helping children deal with procedures.

SUMMARY

Patient education is practiced by using a process of diagnosis and intervention. Motivation and learning theory

TABLE 1-5   Features of Development that are Pertinent to Helping Children Deal with Procedures

	Birth-2 Years	2-7 Years	7-12 Years	Adolescence
How the child thinks and problem solves	Sensory motor experience develops schema (well-defined and repeated sequences of actions and perceptions). Memory is obvious by 3-4 months and is demonstrated in second year by child's imitations of parents' activities. Between about 18 and 24 months, use of symbols for thought-reasoning communication appears.	Preoperational stage (thinking is dominated by the child's perceptions rather than logic). Verbally communicated information is increasingly important in learning; exploratory manipulation of objects also helps the child to learn. Child watches, listens, asks questions (why? how?). Child can (a) label (classify) familiar things; perception is often limited to a single, salient feature, making it difficult for child to see things in a context or differentiate unessential from essential properties of an experience; (b) use memory to reconstruct past events; (c) use imagination to deal with events, people, objects; (d) about age 4 years, begin to infer outcomes; (e) define objects/events in terms of their use/function. Thinking relies on the child's own point of view (egocentricity) because children do not have the capacity to identify a point of view other than their own. As the child gets older, he or she begins to	Concrete operational phase. Child learns from observing/interacting with peers as well as from own experiences. Can use symbols to organize thoughts and represent experience. Features of thinking include increasing capacity to (a) understand viewpoints of others; (b) see the relative nature of things (e.g., this hurts a little; that hurts a lot); (c) use deductive logic in respect to tangible (concrete) experiences (if this, then that); (d) classify things in terms of several characteristics, implying that the child can view things in context, for example, "The shot hurt, but it will make me feel better"; (e) evaluate painful intrusive actions in terms of logical function rather than in terms of punishment; and (f) understand unseen	Stage of formal operations. At this point, there is use of reason and logical thinking and interest in theoretically possible problems and questions. The adolescent can engage in self-reflection and think about own thinking and can learn from verbally presented ideas and arguments.

	be able to think in terms of quantities (e.g., to recognize variation in quantity; to use numbers to count). Attention is increasingly selective as the child's schema or perceptual sets become more refined.	body mechanics/functions. Child can make use of sensory as well as procedural information.	
Major fears and worries	After about 6 months: separation from parents; unfamiliar people/experiences/places, especially when not accompanied by parent	Separation from parents; harm to body, including fears of castration after about age 3 years; punishment for wrongdoing	Body injury; disability (loss of body functions); loss of control; loss of status	Uncertainty about selves as persons (especially early and middle adolescence); concern about whether body, thoughts, and feelings are "normal"
Understanding cause and effect	By about 3 months, may associate an action with a result. In second year: magical thinking: belief that what is wished for happens	Beliefs: (a) everything happens by intention; (b) imminent justice—misbehavior is followed by punishment; (c) belief that events that in fact are associated only by happenstance are connected	Child 6-8 years: conclusions are based on perceptions. Child 9-12 years: applies logical operations (deductive thinking) to concrete (immediately experienced) circumstances. Before about 9 years, children are likely to view their illness as a consequence of transgressions of rules. (Rules exist in their own right and misdeeds have their own inherent punishment.) Before 9 years, children are likely to believe that illness is caused by germs whose presence	Can use formal rules of logic and evidence to assess cause and effect

Continued

TABLE 1-5	Features of Development that are Pertinent to Helping Children Deal with Procedures—cont'd			
	Birth-2 Years	**2-7 Years**	**7-12 Years**	**Adolescence**
Concept of time	By about 3 months, shows anticipation for feedings. Can wait as a consequence of perceiving clues of a familiar and desired activity	Organized around familiar/ routine activities of daily living. By about age 4 years, has concept of time and day and knows days of week	is sufficient for illness. At about 9 years, children begin to understand that (a) an illness may have multiple causes, (b) the body's response to an agent or a combination of agents may vary, and (c) host factors interact with agent(s) to cause illness. Has a concept of the past and future as well as of the present. Can understand time intervals between events and can tell time by a clock. Sense of time is thus more independent of perceptual data (e.g., activities of daily living).	Can synthesize the past, present, and future in thinking
Intentions, goals, and plans	By about 4 months, may show signs of intention/a sense of making an effort to get a result. In second year, child can make a choice of two options.	About age 4 years, begins to plan and anticipate actions in the near future; has objectives for activities	Plans more elaborate projects that involve others to a greater extent	By mid adolescence (about age 15 years), makes future plans for self. Can think in terms of tasks as well as responsibilities in relation to them

Handling emotion	By about 7 months, the child cries for attention, help, or when distressed. By about 9 months, begins to express fears (e.g., separation) in play	Expresses emotion through motor responses and through play. Learns to label feelings. Needs trusted adult to reassure, set limits, prevent loss of self-control	Has a greater capacity to express emotion in verbal terms; can describe fears. Can use projective methods to describe fears (e.g., explain how another child might feel or respond in a specific situation)	May use a range of modalities, from relatively sophisticated verbal or written expression to motor activity and, perhaps, regressed ways of behaving. Thoughts, feelings, and fears may be shared with friends, especially peers. By mid adolescence, has begun to learn how to negotiate a relationship with a clinician
Relationship with parent/clinicians	Developing a sense of self/others. In latter half of first year, beginning to sustain the memory of parent in parent's absence, at least for a short time. Depends on adult to know child's wants/needs	Child is likely to have had experience in relating needs and worries to daycare or church school teachers or clinicians. Children may not expect clinicians to perceive/understand how they feel about things until about the age of 10 years.	May test limits set by caretaker/clinician	
Self-evaluation	Feelings about self are derived from feeling tones communicated by others and perceived by the child.	Develops expectations of self; learns to inhibit own actions. Begins to use other children as models	Evaluates self in terms of performance relative to that of peers and in relation to the set of norms that children believe to be predetermined for them	May use a set of criteria consciously adopted to evaluate self

From Pridham KF, Adelson F, Hansen MF: Helping children deal with procedures in a clinic setting: a developmental approach. *J Pediatr Nurs* 2:13-22, 1987.

provide the base that is needed to plan and to be successful in teaching. Learners are motivated by helping them set their own goals, expressing clear feedback about what they did right, providing effective praise and removing barriers to action. Motivational interviewing is an interesting new approach, as yet unproved for use in chronic diseases. Individual differ-ences in self-directedness, failure tolerance, attributional style, past experience with the task, and expectation of success influence choices to engage and persist in learning. Learning theory, research about kinds of learning, developmental phases, and cultural traditions describe conditions understood to be necessary in changing to a new state of understanding or behavior that persists.

Study Questions

1. It has been said that patients seek help when they are no longer able to cope with their problems at their current level of under-standing. If this statement is at least partly true, what are the implications for health care services?
2. List the questions that you would ask to assess need and motivation to learn in each of the following clinical situations.
   a. You are to teach breast self-examination to groups of women in the waiting room of a gynecology clinic.
   b. You are to teach a 10-year-old boy with cerebral palsy who is mentally disabled and blind how to feed himself.
3. Because an increasing number of high-risk infants are discharged to home with complex medical needs, parents are receiving instruc-tion in cardiopulmonary resuscitation (CPR). One study[21] showed that parents lost informa-tion over time and that those who were regularly reinforced with hands-on demonstra-tion during clinic visits retained the most skills. Are you surprised by the findings? What learning principles were used?
4. Pelco and others[22] describes an approach to teaching a 4-year-old girl how to take a capsule, using behavioral learning principles. Label the behavioral approaches being used.

Teaching Action	Behavioral Approach
a. Child refused to accept any capsules.	
b. Therapist showed child how to swallow by putting capsule between his fingers, placing it on back of his tongue, taking a sip of juice, tilting his head, and swallowing.	
c. Explained to child that by doing what therapist asked, she could earn pennies to buy toys displayed in the room.	
d. When child refused to swallow, therapist placed his hand over child's and guided it through the steps, until she successfully swallowed capsule.	
e. Pennies and praise were given even if physical guidance was used and child swallowed smaller capsule. These steps were followed until child could consistently swallow prescription-sized capsules. Parent was trained how to maintain routine capsule acceptance postintervention.	

REFERENCES

1. Adamian MS, Golin CE, Shain LS, DeVellis B: Brief motivational interviewing to improve adherence to anti-retroviral therapy: development and qualitative pilot assessment of an intervention. *AIDS Pat Care & STDs* 18:229-238, 2004.

2. Akimoto M and others: Psychosocial predictors of relapse among diabetes patients: a 2-year follow-up after inpatient diabetes education. *Psychomatics* 45:343-349, 2004.

3. Bandura A: Self-efficacy mechanism in human agency. *Am Psychol* 37:122-147, 1982.

4. Bandura A: *Foundations of thought and action: a social cognitive theory*, Englewood Cliffs, NJ, 1986, Prentice-Hall.

5. Bandura A: *Self efficacy; the exercise of control*, New York, 1997, Freeman.

6. Benavides-Vaello S, Garcia AA, Brown SA, Winchell M: Using focus groups to plan and evaluate diabetes self-management interventions for Mexican Americans. *Diab Educ* 30:238-256, 2004.

7. Britt E, Hudson SM, Blampied NM: Motivational interviewing in health settings: a review. *Paient Educ Counsel* 53:147-155, 2004.

8. Bucher JA and others: Problem-solving cancer care education for patients and caregivers. *Canc Pract* 9:66-70, 2001.

9. Carino JL, Coke L, Gulanick M: Using motivational interviewing to reduce diabetes risk. *Prog Cardiovasc Nurs* 19:149-154, 2004.

10. Elkind D: Teenage thinking: implications for health care. *Pediatr Nurs* 10:383-385, 1984.

11. Glaser R, Bassok M: Learning theory and the study of instruction. *Annu Rev Psychol* 40:631-666, 1989.

12. Guzman SJ, Nicassio PM: The contributions of negative and positive illness schemas to depression in patients with end-stage renal disease. *J Behav Med* 26:517-534, 2003.

13. Horne R: Representations of medications and treatment. In Petrie KJ, Weinman JA, editors: *Perceptions of health and illness*, Amsterdam, 1997, Harwood Academic Press.

14. Jonassen DH, Peck KL, Wilson BG: *Learning with technology; a constructivist perspective*, Columbus, Ohio, 1999, Merrill Press.

15. Kloeblen AS, Batish SS: Understanding the intention to permanently follow a high folate diet among a sample of low-income pregnant women according to the Health Belief Model, *Health Educ Res* 14:327-338, 1999.

16. Lewis FM, Daltroy LH: How causal explanations influence health behavior: attribution theory. In Glanz K, Lewis FM, Rimer BK, editors: *Health behavior and health education*, San Francisco, 1990, Jossey-Bass.

17. Ley P: Memory for medical information, *Br J Soc Clin Psychol* 18:245-255, 1979.

18. Mezirow J: *Transformative learning*, San Francisco, 1991, Jossey-Bass.

19. Miller SM: Monitoring versus blunting styles of coping with cancer influence the information patients want and need about their disease. *Cancer* 76:167-177, 1995.

20. Mullen PD, Hersey JC, Iverson DC: Health behavior models compared. *Soc Sci Med* 24:973-981, 1987.

21. Paul S, Sneed NV: Strategies for behavior change in patients with heart failure. *Am J Crit Care* 13:305-313, 2004.

22. Pelco LE and others: Behavioral management of oral medication administration difficulties among children: a review of literature with case illustration, *J Dev Behav Pediatr* 8:90-96, 1987.

23. Pestrak VA, Martin D: Cognitive development and aspects of adolescent sexuality, *Adolescence* 20:981-987, 1985.

24. Peterson KA, Hughes M: Readiness to change and clinical success in a diabetes educational program. *JABFP* 15:266-271, 2002.

25. Pridham KF, Adelson F, Hansen MF: Helping children deal with procedures in a clinic setting: a developmental approach. *J Pediatr Nurs* 2:13-22, 1987.

26. Prochaska JO and others: The transtheoretical model of change and HIV prevention: a review. *Health Educ Q* 21:471-486, 1994.

27. Rosenstock IM, Strecher VJ, Becker MH: The health belief model and HIV risk behavior change. In Di Clemente RJ, Peterson JL, editors: *Preventing AIDS: theories and methods of behavioral interventions*, New York, 1994, Plenum Press.

28. Ryan RM, Deci EL: Self-determination theory and the facilitation of intrinsic motivation, social development, and well-being. *Am Psychol* 55:68-78, 2000.

29. Salomon G, Perkins DN: Rocky roads to transfer: rethinking mechanisms of a neglected phenomenon. *Educ Psychol* 24:113-142, 1989.

30. Schorloo M, Kaptein A: Measurement of illness perceptions in patients with chronic somatic illnesses: a review. In Petrie KJ, Weinman JA, editors: *Perceptions of health and illness*, Amsterdam, 1997, Harwood Academic Press.

31. Slavin RE: *Educational psychology: theory into practice*, Englewood Cliffs, NJ, 1994, Prentice-Hall.

32. Taylor EW: Building upon the theoretical debate: a critical review of the empirical studies of Mezirow's transformative learning theory. *Adult Educ Quart* 48:34-59, 1997.

33. Van Merrienboer JG, Kirschner PA, Kester L: Taking the load off a learner's mind: instructional design for complex learning. *Educ Psychol* 38:5-13, 2003.

34. Wiginton KL: Illness representations: mapping the experience of lupus. *Health Educ Behav* 26:443-453, 1999.

35. Woolfolk A: *Educational psychology*, 8th ed., Boston, 2001, Allyn & Bacon.

2

Educational Objectives and Instruction

EDUCATIONAL OBJECTIVES

Statements of goals and objectives are intended learning outcomes. They provide direction for choosing instructional activities that will yield those outcomes.

Constructivist philosophies of learning suggest that patients should set their own goals and priorities and learn in "real" settings. Such an approach aims to avoid production of inert knowledge that is difficult to apply or transfer to meaningful contexts. Under this philosophy, specific learning objectives should be set, at least in part, by the learner. A study of patients with diabetes shows that they need a certain level of education before they are able to set specific objectives without leaving serious knowledge gaps that could affect self-management.[11]

A statement of objectives requires the use of terms with precise meanings congruent with the appropriate level of outcome (Box 2-1), and a statement of both a behavior and a content. Knowledge is the lowest level of intellectual outcome and is concerned with recall or recognition of learned material. Comprehension is concerned with grasping the meaning of material as shown by interpretation, translation, prediction, and similar responses. Application is the ability to use the material in new situations.[23] The objectives flowing from the situation described in Box 2-2 demonstrate these characteristics.

INSTRUCTIONAL FORMS

Instruction is designed to ensure conditions that support learning. The following summary highlights the guidelines from motivation and learning introduced in the first chapter[34]:

- Begin with objectives, including patients' objectives, and keep them in focus from planning through evaluation.
- Design instruction according to patients' abilities, knowledge structures, and expectations.
- Provide realistic tasks that patients can become competent at performing and believe that they can perform competently.
- Provide advance organizers to constitute "ideational scaffolding" (a structure of ideas) in learning. These statements summarize the

Box 2-1	*Types of Learning Outcomes Common to Many Areas and Levels of Instruction*

Lower-Level Cognitive
   Outcomes
   Knowledge
   Comprehension
   Application
{
Recalling
Translating
Interpreting
Estimating
Comparing
Classifying
Applying

Higher-Level Thinking Skills
   Analysis
   Synthesis
   Evaluation
{
Identifying
Analyzing
Inferring
Relating
Formulating
Generating
Judging

Affective Outcomes
   Attitudes
   Interests
   Appreciations
   Adjustments
{
Listening
Responding
Participating
Seeking
Demonstrating
Relating
Valuing

Performance Outcomes
   Procedure
   Product
   Procedure and product
   Problem solving
{
Speaking
Singing
Drawing
Computing
Writing
Constructing
Demonstrating
Operating
Performing
Originating

From Gronlund NE: *Writing instructional objectives for teaching and assessment*, ed 7, Upper Saddle River, NJ, 2004, Pearson Merrill Prentice Hall. Reprinted with permission.

Box 2-2	*Statement of Objectives*

Situation

A home health nurse is teaching a wife and a daughter how to care for a bedfast elderly husband and father. The patient moves little but has not been incontinent. He has had no skin breakdown yet but, according to the wife, has been allowed to lie in one position for 4 hours. The main objective is part of the more encompassing objective, to avoid the harmful consequences of bedrest.

Main Objective

To avoid pressure ulcer formation (psychomotor, cognitive, affective)

Subobjectives

A. To recognize any evidence of tissue breakdown by inspecting at least once a day (cognitive, comprehension; psychomotor, perception)
B. To reposition the patient at least every 2 hours, so that the body is resting on the same surface only every fourth time (psychomotor, mechanism; cognitive, comprehension)
C. To keep all linen wrinkle free (psychomotor, mechanism; cognitive, knowledge)
D. To cleanse skin at the time of soiling and at routine intervals (psychomotor, mechanism; cognitive, comprehension)
E. To report to the nurse evidence of incontinence or skin breakdown within 4 hours after it is observed (cognitive, knowledge)
F. To maintain adequate nutritional intake (cognitive, knowledge)

essence of the lesson and integrate it with previously learned material.
- Provide models with whom patients identify and from whom they can learn.

- Match instruction to patients' stages of readiness and stimulate readiness when necessary.
- Divide complex tasks into smaller, achievable sequential learning units so that patients can experience satisfaction and a feeling of self-efficacy.
- Organize complex information in easy-to-remember structures such as graphics or schematics.

- Practice instruction in a variety of ways to match different learning styles (oral, visual). Ample learning time should be used for practice that is participatory and experiential and that uses different senses.
- Provide immediate feedback so that patients can improve their responses.
- Conclude instruction by having patients review what they have learned and feel confident they can do and by observing them do it in real-world settings.

Most instructional forms are familiar to readers of this book. They have three basic components: (1) a delivery system, which is the physical form of the materials and hardware used to present stimuli to the learners, such as handouts, slides, computer-assisted instruction, or a person; (2) a content or message; and (3) a form or condition of abstractness. Figure 2-1 shows an example of the abstract-concrete continuum. Methods are also instructor centered, interactive, individualized, or experiential (Table 2-1).

Patient education also fits within taxonomies of interventions describing the practice of particular professions. One of the several taxonomies for nursing is the Nursing Intervention Classification Project, which describes patient education as one class of intervention within the behavioral domain. The project describes more than 400 nursing interventions categorized into classes and domains.[26] This work creates a standardized language for nursing treatments. More specific "intervention labels" related to patient education include participatory guidance, decision-making support, learning facilitation, childbirth preparation, learning-readiness enhancement, parent education, preparatory sensory information, teaching: disease process, teaching: group, teaching: individual, teaching: infant care, teaching: preoperative, teaching: prescribed activity/exercise, teaching: prescribed diet, teaching: prescribed medication, teaching: procedure/treatment, teaching: psychomotor skill, and teaching: safe sex. Box 2-3 shows one of the teaching interventions with its definition and activities. This class of teaching interventions is among those with the highest use among practicing nurses.[8]

Interpersonal Teaching Forms

Probably the most potent learning occurs experientially in real situations, by patients making the judgments and doing the tasks they will need to do for themselves, directed by their sense of need to become competent. Learning from peers who have successfully completed the transition on which patients are embarking often provides models and an emotional identification that is motivating. Such conditions integrate cognitive, affective, and psychomotor learning in a single performance. These conditions must be reconstructed as a patient enters a new phase of readjustment and faces new challenges and goals. Because education has traditionally been delivered in settings in which highly technical health care is provided, learning conditions realistic to everyday life have been considerably underused. When patient education is taken seriously, realistic, experiential learning environments are created and tested. Considerable evidence shows that, with a patient's mastering of a basic knowledge base, these realistic, motivating, learning environments will be the most effective of the methods

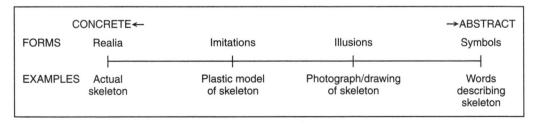

FIGURE 2-1 Form of instructional materials: the abstract-concrete continuum. (Modified from Weston C, Cranton PA: Selecting instructional strategies, *J Higher Educ* 57:259-288, 1986.)

TABLE 2-1	**Summary of Instructional Methods**		
INSTRUCTOR-CENTERED	**INTERACTIVE**	**INDIVIDUALIZED**	**EXPERIENTIAL**
Lecture	**Class Discussion**	**Programmed Instruction**	**Field or Clinical**
Passive students Efficient for lower learning levels and large classes	Must have small class size May be time consuming Encourages student involvement	Most effective at lower learning levels Very structured Allows students to work at own pace Extensive feedback for students	Occurs in natural setting during performance Active student involvement May be difficult for management and evaluation
Questioning	**Discussion Groups**	**Modularized Instruction**	**Laboratory**
Monitors student learning Encourages student involvement May cause anxiety for some	Small class size Student participation Effective for high cognitive and affective learning levels	May be time consuming Very flexible formats Allows students to work at own pace	Requires careful planning and evaluation Active student involvement in realistic setting
Demonstration	**Peer Teaching**	**Independent Projects**	**Role Playing**
Illustrates an application of a skill or concept Students are passive	Requires careful planning and monitoring Uses differences in student expertise Encourages student involvement	Most appropriate at higher learning levels May be time consuming Active student involvement in learning	Effective in affective and psychomotor domains Provides "safe" experiences Active student participation
	Group Projects	**Computerized Instruction**	**Simulations and Games**
	Requires careful planning and monitoring Uses differences in student expertise Encourages student involvement	May involve considerable instructor time or expense May be very flexible Allows students to work at own pace Student involvement in varying activities	Provide practice of specific skills Produce anxiety for some Active student participation **Drill** Most appropriate at lower learning levels Provides active practice May not be motivating for some students

Modified from Weston C, Cranton PA: Selecting instructional strategies, *J Higher Educ* 57:259-288, 1986.

Box 2-3	*Teaching: Prescribed Diet*

Definition

Preparing a patient to correctly follow a prescribed diet

Activities

Appraise the patient's current level of knowledge about the prescribed diet.

Determine the patient's/significant other's feelings/attitude toward the prescribed diet and expected degree of dietary compliance.

Inform the patient of the proper name of the prescribed diet.

Explain the purpose of the diet.

Inform the patient how long the diet should be followed.

Instruct the patient how to keep a food diary as appropriate.

Instruct the patient on allowed and prohibited foods.

Inform the patient of possible drug/food interactions as appropriate.

Assist the patient to accommodate food preferences into the prescribed diet.

Assist the patient in substituting ingredients to conform favorite recipes to the prescribed diet.

Instruct the patient how to read labels and select appropriate foods.

Observe the patient's selection of foods appropriate to the prescribed diet.

Instruct the patient how to plan appropriate meals.

Provide written meal plans as appropriate.

Recommend a cookbook that includes recipes consistent with prescribed diet as appropriate.

Reinforce information provided by other health care team members as appropriate.

Refer patient to dietitian/nutritionist as appropriate.

Include the family/significant others as appropriate.

From McCloskey Dochterman JC, Bulechek GM, editors: *Nursing interventions classifications (NIC)*, ed 4, St Louis, 2004, Mosby.

known, even for patients with little formal education.

Groups provide an economical way to teach. The experience of having the support of a group, gaining motivation to learn from other members, decreasing feelings of isolation, and modeling the behavior of other individuals may be the best way for patients to meet their objectives.

For example, caregivers of persons with Alzheimer's disease and related disorders need groups that focus on education and support. Such help is necessary because of the progressive deterioration of the patient's condition over a 7- to 10-year period. Experiences include role reversals, little support from peers or other family members, absent or misinterpreted feedback from the patient, and withdrawal from social networks. These unpleasant changes can result in progressive deterioration of the family system and in depression for caregivers. Caregivers can learn specific skills, such as how to respond to the patient's behavior and cognitive impairments, how to modify his or her environment, and how to deal with legal and financial problems, sadness, frustration, and anger. It is less expensive for the family to be involved in effective educational and support groups than it is to institutionalize the patient if the caregiver fails to cope. One study of caregivers for frail elderly persons in the community finds that the institutionalization rate decreases from 17% to 5% when the caregivers are involved in educational or support groups. The educational program focused on assisting caregivers in dealing constructively with negative feelings, as well as on how to lift, move, and bathe the patient and how to administer medication. Social skills for dealing with the patient and other family members and relaxation techniques were also taught. The availability of a secondary caregiver was important.[22]

Annually, 6.4 million people participate in member-governed, problem-specific, low-fee self-help groups. Health professionals are involved with these groups in various ways but usually are not central to them. Some groups are small and local; others are nationally networked assemblies. Members are psychologically bonded by the compelling similarity of their concerns. They rely primarily on the collective experiential knowledge possessed by the membership. Acceptance by the group seems to be a vital step toward making the cognitive, emotional, and behavioral changes necessary for more effective functioning and an improved quality of life. One database in California found 188 distinct problem categories around which groups were formed. Support groups address problems such as alcoholism, anorexia, arthritis, parental bereavement, coping with various cancers, care taking of persons with Alzheimer's disease, diabetes, burns, drug abuse, impact of incest, and parental coping with handicapped children, as well as many others.[27]

Some groups form spontaneously. In one case, informal support groups were evolving as patients with ventricular tachycardia, who were in a hospital for electrophysiological studies and treatment, socialized in their rooms and in the lounge. The disadvantage of this development was that misinformation was easily passed on. Because the disease was life threatening and the treatment invasive, the disruption caused by misinformation could have been serious. A formal program was therefore developed with a teaching component that included information on normal electrical conduction in the heart and the pathology of ventricular tachycardia, electrophysiological studies, telemetry monitoring, medications, and preparation for discharge.

Certification in cardiopulmonary resuscitation for family members and friends was also offered. Patients exhibiting severe anxiety, frank denial, or overt hostility were screened out of the group and taught individually.[14]

In another example, Kulik and Mahler[30] describe groups that formed even when it was not intended. Patients whose roommates had already had surgery before their own operations were less anxious preoperatively, they were more ambulatory postoperatively, and they were released 1.4 days more quickly than were patients whose roommates also had not had surgery yet. Social comparison theory predicts that evaluative needs of individuals in unusual and stressful situations are best served by comparison with others who are in similar situations. Roommates' experiences may also provide patients with information preoperatively that will enable them to interpret postoperative sensations and events in a more accurate and less personally threatening manner. With today's brief preoperative stays, such opportunities may no longer exist.

Sometimes it is important to form separate groups for patients and for families. It is also useful to prescreen individuals entering a group to assess whether their learning needs are generally the same or whether one individual would be disruptive to the group. Group appointments, in which patients and others with the same diagnosis are seen by a multidisciplinary team for extended visits, are gaining popularity in managed care settings.

Figure 2-2 describes a contingency contract between patient and provider. Desired behaviors, rewards, punishments, and time frames are discussed, written and signed by the patient. Research shows that these contracts yield at least short-term, positive effects across a variety of medication and health-related behaviors. However, long-term results show considerable recidivism.[28]

Role Playing

Role playing is an excellent technique for diagnosis of motivation and readiness to learn, as well as for teaching ideas and attitudes. People are assigned to play themselves or someone else. A related technique is for the teacher to enact a

Date

Heath-care contract

Contract goal: (Specific outcome to be attained)

I, (client's name), agree to (detailed description of required behaviors, time and frequency limitations)

in return for (positive reinforcements contingent upon completion of required behaviors; timing and mode of delivery of reinforcements)

I, (provider's name), agree to (detailed description of required behaviors, time and frequency limitations)

(Optional) I, (significant other's name), agree to (detailed description of required behaviors, time and frequency limitations)

(Optional) Aversive consequences: (Negative reinforcements for failure to meet minimum behavioral requirements)

(Optional) Bonuses: (Additional positive reinforcements for exceeding minimum contract requirements)

We will review the terms of this agreement and will make any desired modifications, on (date). We hereby agree to abide by the terms of the contract described above.

Signed: (Client) _____
Signed: (Significant other, if relevant)

_____

Signed: (Provider) _____
Contract effective from (Date) _____
to (Date) _____

FIGURE 2-2 Patient-provider contingency contract. (From Janz NK, Becker MH, Hartman PE: Contingency contracting to enhance patient compliance: a review, *Patient Educ Couns* 5:164-178, 1984.)

role that the learner can model. For example, the teacher could enact a positive or desirable parental role in relation to a child's specific behavior and then discuss and label the behavior that has been portrayed.

Through role playing, a desired behavior is rehearsed. Thus a person is taught the skills required and gains the confidence needed to carry them out. Reversal of roles is a technique useful for sensitizing one person to the other's situation. Role playing provides a kind of behavioral and mental rehearsal that is a form of practice. It is also a means of increasing retention in learning.

Role playing techniques have been cited as useful in teaching persons from disadvantaged backgrounds. These techniques are effective in situations that have been described as physical, action oriented, concrete, and problem directed rather than those that are introspective. They are most effective when instruction is easy and informally paced. Role playing may also reduce the role distance between patient and professional. The technique has considerable potential for reducing overintellectualization and for uniting understanding and feeling.

For all these reasons, school-aged children are often taught how to deal with their asthma by using puppets to role-play. At this stage of child development, the chief learning mode is visual and psychomotor (puppets), and teachers focus on helping the children develop an "I can do" attitude (role playing). Box 2-4 contains suggested role-playing situations with use of puppets. The role playing is designed to help children manage an asthma attack, take their medications correctly, and cope with teasing from peers.

Role playing is often incorporated as one technique in a program. For example, one educationally oriented support group for teenagers with diabetes began with a weekend camping

Box 2-4	*Suggested Role Play Situations*

Lesson 1

Wheezing Willie is very allergic to grass. If he is near it, he will wheeze and may even have an asthma attack. He is at his friend's house for a birthday party and the children decide to do somersaults and cartwheels on the freshly cut grass. What should Wheezing Willie do?

Lesson 2

Healthy Heather has been given the assignment to tell the class what happens to the human body when it has an asthma attack.

Lesson 3

Wheezing Wendy and her family have just moved to a new neighborhood and she is going to a new school. In the morning of her first day, she begins to wheeze. The person sitting next to her hears her wheezing and starts to call her names. What should Wheezing Wendy do?

Lesson 4

Wheezing Willie has to take a breathing treatment and other medication every day at school during the lunch period. Because he has to take a treatment, he misses half of recess. Lately, Willie has been feeling well and has stopped going to the office to take his breathing treatment and medication. Do you think Wheezing Willie is doing the right thing? What should he do?

Lesson 5

Wheezing Wendy is at her friend Healthy Heather's house. She is having fun playing with Barbie dolls when she begins to have a headache and her throat starts to feel scratchy. These are two of Wheezing Wendy's early warning signs. Wheezing Wendy's mother is at work and won't be home for 2 more hours. What should she do?

From Ramsey AM, Siroky AS: The use of puppets to teach school-age children with asthma, *Pediatr Nurs* 14:187-190, 1988.

experience to bond the group. The group members wore identical T-shirts with a logo to aid in group identity. The members quickly discovered that the group was a place to meet with friends. Role playing on how to relate to parents and other family members was a critical element of the program. Snacks were cooked, and awards were given for each teenager's special trait. Blood glucose was tested before and after exercise. The teenagers gained experience in solving actual problems, and they signed contracts agreeing to certain future behaviors.[12]

Demonstration and Practice

Demonstration is a performance of procedures or psychomotor skills, which, combined with practice, is the method most suited to attaining skills. The purpose of the demonstration is to give the learner a clear mental image of how the procedure is performed. Presentations of a prime view by video may be necessary if the groups are large. In some instances an over-the-shoulder view of the demonstrator provides learners with a clear idea of the way they must perform the action. When the demonstrator is removing fluids from a vial and giving an injection, the mirror image that viewers receive by facing the demonstrator is not entirely realistic.

Learners need practice to develop motor skills; therefore, the teaching plan must incorporate a time for patients to practice. When equipment is sufficient and the group is small enough, practice may begin with the learner demonstrating the skill immediately after the teacher finishes. Additional practice should take place in a setting similar to that in which the skill will be used. The teacher must supervise enough to provide feedback for correct performance and to stimulate motivation if necessary.

Teaching Tools

Much teaching is accomplished by means of tools, both written and audiovisual, used within the context of an instructional plan. If these tools are well designed and have been shown to be effective in creating learning, and if they are well matched to the goals of instruction and to the learner's capabilities, they can be almost self-instructional.

Written materials are by far the most frequently used in patient education, despite persistent evidence that they are mismatched to the needs of many patients, particularly in their reading level. Printed teaching material can be described as a frozen language that is selective in its description of reality (which is both a strength and a weakness). It encourages limited feedback but is constantly available. Print partially relaxes time requirements and is more efficient than oral language (except for those who have not learned to read efficiently) because readers can control the speed at which they read and comprehend. Certain kinds of thinking seem to demand written expression. For example, a complex sequence of thoughts that incorporates definitions, qualifications, and logical constraints is expressed best in writing. Most people who have learned to read well generally prefer to acquire information by reading. Reading is ideal for understanding complex concepts and relationships. If the learning objective primarily requires skill in dealing with persons or things, then demonstrations, concrete experience with the activity, and oral coaching and guidance would be more effective than print media.

The various media that can be used for learning possess cognitively relevant characteristics in their technologies, symbol systems, and processing capabilities. Computers are distinguished by their extensive processing capabilities rather than by their access to a particularly unique set of symbol systems (they use words and pictures) and by the wide and frequently confusing variety of materials of varying quality on the internet. On video, the symbols can depict action; however, the symbols are transient.[19]

Although some students can learn a particular task regardless of the medium, others need the advantage of a particular medium's characteristics. For example, experts who learn from text can skim rapidly, using trigger words to read selectively and nonsequentially. When memory limits are reached, they stop and summarize the material they have learned. Such processing

strategies cannot be used with audiotapes or lectures. Novices take advantage of the text's stability to slow the rate of information processing; as a result, they are able to review the material. Pictures that illustrate information central to the text help the reader. If, however, the material is too difficult for the reader, he or she must expend a great deal of effort trying to decode the text, possibly increasing the risk of learning failure.[29]

Print Materials

Because different media have different strengths, use of a variety of media is likely to be more successful than is use of a single medium. Learning from print materials is an economical use of time, if they are well designed to promote learning and if they match a patient's reading and literacy levels. Approximately half the population in the United States struggles with basic reading skills. For many others the materials available are written at a higher level than they can comprehend. The reading levels of many individuals may be up to five grades below the grade they report to have completed.

Graphic design techniques that can increase readership, comprehension, and memory are summarized in Box 2-5.[9] For low-literacy readers, increase the amount of white space and use a question and answer or bullet (not paragraph) format.[34] Photographs and illustrations decrease the density of the text. In addition, authors of print materials should do the following:

- Make key messages easy to find.
- Use the first paragraph to communicate the benefits the audience desires most and the actions to obtain them.
- Provide true or fictional stories about people taking concrete actions and experiencing consequences that are interesting to the audience.
- Describe step-by-step the action requested.
- Provide pictures and words that evoke vivid imagery, which will be better remembered than abstract words.
- Write text in second person to convey information personally relevant to readers.

Box 2-5	*Graphic Design Guidelines for Easy-to-Read and Effective Written Materials*

To Direct Readers to the Message

Do	Don't
• Use arrows, underlines, bold type, boxes, white space, and bullets to direct readers' eyes to the key messages.	• Use italics, all capital letters, script, or screens of color over text. • Require reader to look in many directions on the page to read copy and find the message.

To Select an Easy-to-Read Typeface

Do	Don't
• Use 10- to 14-point type size. • Use a typeface with serifs in the body copy (e.g., Times Roman).	• Go below 10-point type size for good readers and 12-point for poor readers. • Mix typefaces or use more than three sizes of print on one page. • Use white letters on black background.

To Create Easy-to-Read Copy

Do	Don't
• Use 40- to 50-character-wide columns, left justified. • Use lots of white space. • Use highly contrasting colors for text and background such as black on white or cream. • Use the same dark color for headings and body copy or colors with similar intensity.	• Break margins with illustrations or other graphics. If required, break only the right margin. • Use light or unusual ink colors such as red, green, or orange.

To Create Clear Visuals

Do	Don't
• Convey one key message per visual. Print the message in a caption. • Make the message easy to grasp at a glance. • Show only the "desired" way to act in visuals. • Use realistic drawings, photos, or human-like figures. • Use visuals with which the audience can identify.	• Add any visuals simply to decorate the material. • Include any details or background in the visual that are not required to communicate the message. • Use highly stylized or abstract graphics. • Portray blood cells and other body parts as cartoon characters.

From Buxton T: Effective ways to improve health education materials, *J Health Educ* 30:47-50, 61, 1999.

- Increase rehearsal of information by repeating it, highlighting it, or boxing it, and ask readers to perform specific activities.
- Provide materials sensitive to the culture of those with whom they will be used, addressing their lifestyles and using cultural language and symbols.

For example, an assessment of prostate cancer patient education materials found them factually accurate but omitting important information. Fewer than half the pamphlets that covered diagnosis discussed what is meant by positive or negative biopsy results and only one discussed the risks of prostate biopsy. Discussion of side effects was incomplete for treatments such as radical prostatectomy, androgen ablation, and radiation therapy.[41]

A spiritually based breast cancer educational booklet for African American women was developed with an advisory panel from the church, for cultural appropriateness and more effective communication.[24] Spiritual themes and scripture were used to frame the early detection messages: the body is a temple of God and a gift to be taken care of and respected; the mammogram will "go easier" when one is calmed by faith.

Of the plethora of studies on readability, most come to the conclusion that many persons who must use written patient education materials have limited ability to understand those that are available.

- Reading grade levels of patient education handouts for 15 of the most frequently prescribed psychotropic drugs in a state mental health facility were at the twelfth to fourteenth grade level, well above the eighth grade level for the general public and the recommended third to fifth grade reading level for low-literacy readers.[36]
- Mean readability of 100 patient pamphlets developed by the American College of Obstetricians and Gynecologists was seventh to ninth grade level. Because the average reading level of U.S. citizens is eighth grade and one in five adults reads at the fifth grade level or below, these materials are also mismatched with many of their intended users.[17]
- On average, patient material on the World Wide Web is written at tenth grade reading level.[20]

The term "readability" refers to the understandabilitiy of written text. It is important to note that readability formulas indicate reading ease, not comprehension, although when the reading level is beyond the skill of the learner, comprehension is known to be decreased and recall is sketchy and inaccurate. There are more than 40 different formulas used to determine readability. Nearly all word processing programs will produce readability statistics, frequently under "tools." In contrast to the amount of attention devoted to measuring readability of materials, little attention has been paid to measuring patient comprehension of, or learning from, educational literature. Other characteristics not captured in readability formulas are also important in written and other instructional materials. These include organization, including use of headings and outlines, appropriate sequencing of material, and clarity. An example of materials written at high levels and revised to be read at much lower levels can be found in Box 2-6.

Literacy

Although readability formulas are used to analyze text, tests of reading ability are administered to individuals for the purpose of selecting appropriate teaching interventions. Of the available tests that have been commonly used in clinical settings, two are health specific. Table 2-2 describes the tests.[32] Signed informed consent before use of these tests may be required because this information may be embarrassing or be used in a biased way if confidentiality is broken. Results should not be recorded in medical charts. The tests can also be used in populations to identify the kinds of educational materials they could use.

Because functional literacy varies by context and setting, tests specific to health are likely to be more useful. Health literacy encompasses a constellation of skills including the ability to perform basic reading and numeracy tasks required to function in the health environment. Interest in it is sparked in part by the fact that health professionals and institutions have liability for adverse

Box 2-6	*Example of Patient Education Materials for Hyperphosphatemia*

Difficult (12th Grade Reading Level):

The patient should be taking phosphorus-binding medications with every meal or snack because these drugs prevent absorption of phosphorus from the gastrointestinal tract into the bloodstream. The excess phosphate eventually leaches calcium from the bones, resulting in weakening of the bone structure.

Easier (5th Grade Reading Level):

You should take some medicines every time you eat a meal or snack. We call these medicines *phosphate binders*. The medicines keep the phosphate in your intestines. This helps calcium stay in your bones and keeps your bones strong and healthy.

From Aldridge MD: Writing and designing readable patient education materials, *Nephrol Nurs J* 31:373-377, 2004. Reprinted with permission of the American Nephrology Nurses Association, publisher.

TABLE 2-2	**Formal Literacy Screening Tests**

Test	Description	Advantages	Disadvantages
TOFHLA			
(Test of Functional Health Literacy in Adults)	50-item comprehension and 17-item numerical ability test based on tasks often required of patients seeking health care (e.g., reading prescription bottle or appointment slip)	Only test that evaluates numerical skills Soon available in Spanish Assesses comprehension, not just word recognition	Not validated prospectively Not available for clinical use
WRAT-R			
(Wide Range Achievement Test-Revised)	Reading recognition test	Takes 3-5 min More accurate than REALM in assessing degree of impairment	Not available in Spanish
SORT-R			
(Slosson Oral Reading Test-Revised)	Measures ability to pronounce words of varying difficulty	Easy to administer and score	Patients dislike the small print and large number of items

Continued

TABLE 2-2	Formal Literacy Screening Tests—cont'd		
Test	**Description**	**Advantages**	**Disadvantages**
	PIAT-R		
(Peabody Individual Achievement Test-Revised)	Reading comprehension subset consists of 88 items. Patients read a sentence and choose from among 4 pictures the one that best represents the meaning of the task.	Assesses comprehension rather than word recognition	Long, takes 30-40 min to complete
	REALM		
(Rapid Estimate of Adult Literacy in Medicine)	Reading recognition test that measures patients' ability to pronounce medical terms. This 66-item version is still valid; much faster than 125-item version. Patients read as many words aloud as possible. Words correctly pronounced scored as plus, nonattempted words scored as minus, and incorrectly pronounced ones as a check.	Items in test relevant to medicine Takes 3-5 min	Spanish version not valid

From Lasater L, Mehler PS: The illiterate patient: screening and management, *Hosp Pract* 33:163-170, 1998.

outcomes of patients who do not understand important health information. Literacy is not only a reading problem; because of limited vocabulary or difficulty following complex sentence structure, these patients are also likely to struggle with oral communication.

Further information on the Test of Functional Health Literacy in Adults (TOFHLA) may be obtained from Nurss and others.[37] It measures comprehension skills in the middle to low levels of literacy ability and takes up to 22 minutes to administer. TOFHLA incorporates common health tasks such as reading prescription vials, interpreting an appointment slip, using a chart describing eligibility for financial aid, understanding results from medical tests, following instructions for an upper gastrointestinal tract test, understanding the patient rights and responsibilities section of a

Medicaid application form, and comprehending a standard hospital informed consent form. Baker and others[3] found that 19% of high school graduates in their study showed inadequate literacy and 11% marginal literacy as measured by TOFHLA. These patients were seeking medical care in the walk-in clinic of an emergency department.

Rapid Estimate of Adult Literacy in Medicine (REALM) is a 66-word reading recognition test that can be used to screen for low literacy in a few minutes. The word list and directions for administering and scoring may be found in Figure 2-3.[13]

One in five adult Americans is functionally illiterate, reading at or below the fifth grade level. Concentrated in inner-city populations, in minorities and among those older than 65 years of age, these individuals understand little if any of the

RAPID ESTIMATE OF ADULT LITERACY IN MEDICINE
(REALM)©

Terry Davis, PhD • Michael Crouch, MD • Sandy Long, PhD

Reading
Level _____

Patient Name/
Subject # _____   Date of Birth _____   Grade
Completed _____

Date _____   Clinic _____   Examiner _____

List 1		List 2		List 3	
fat	_____	fatigue	_____	allergic	_____
flu	_____	pelvic	_____	menstrual	_____
pill	_____	jaundice	_____	testicle	_____
dose	_____	infection	_____	colitis	_____
eye	_____	exercise	_____	emergency	_____
stress	_____	behavior	_____	medication	_____
smear	_____	prescription	_____	occupation	_____
nerves	_____	notify	_____	sexually	_____
germs	_____	gallbladder	_____	alcoholism	_____
meals	_____	calories	_____	irritation	_____
disease	_____	depression	_____	constipation	_____
cancer	_____	miscarriage	_____	gonorrhea	_____
caffeine	_____	pregnancy	_____	inflammatory	_____
attack	_____	arthritis	_____	diabetes	_____
kidney	_____	nutrition	_____	hepatitis	_____
hormones	_____	menopause	_____	antibiotics	_____
herpes	_____	appendix	_____	diagnosis	_____
seizure	_____	abnormal	_____	potassium	_____
bowel	_____	syphilis	_____	anemia	_____
asthma	_____	hemorrhoids	_____	obesity	_____
rectal	_____	nausea	_____	osteoporosis	_____
incest	_____	directed	_____	impetigo	_____

SCORE

List 1 _____
List 2 _____
List 3 _____
Raw
Score _____

FIGURE 2-3 Rapid Estimate of Adult Literacy in Medicine (REALM)©. (From Davis TL and others: Practical assessment of adult literacy in health care, *Health Educ Behav* 25:613-624, 1998.)

Continued

RAPID ESTIMATE OF ADULT LITERACY IN MEDICINE

The Rapid Estimate of Adult Literacy in Medicine (REALM) is a screening instrument to assess an adult patient's ability to read common medical words and lay terms for body parts and illnesses. It is designed to assist medical professionals in estimating a patient's literacy level so that the appropriate level of patient education materials or oral instructions may be used. The test takes 2 to 3 minutes to administer and score. The REALM has been correlated with other standardized tests.

	Correlation of REALM with SORT, PIAT-R, and WRAT-R		
	PIAT-R Recognition	SORT	WRAT-R
Correlation Coefficient	.97	.96	.88
P Value	p<.0001	p<.0001	p<.0001

Reliability Studies	
Test-Retest	Inter-Rater
(n = 100)	(n = 20)
.99	.99

DIRECTIONS:

1. Give the patient a laminated copy of the REALM and score answers on an unlaminated copy that is attached to a clipboard. Hold the clipboard at an angle so that the patient is not distracted by your scoring procedure. Say:

    "I want to hear you read as many words as you can from this list. Begin with the first word on List 1 and read aloud. When you come to a word you cannot read, do the best you can or say "blank" and go on to the next word."

2. If the patient takes more than five seconds on a word, say "blank" and point to the next word, if necessary, to move the patient along. If the patient begins to miss every word, have him/her pronounce only known words.

3. Count as an error any word not attempted or mispronounced. Score by marking a plus (+) after each correct word, a check (√) after each mispronounced word, and a minus (−) after words not attempted. Count as correct any self-corrected word.

4. Count the number of correct words for each list and record the numbers in the "SCORE" box. Total the numbers and match the total score with its grade equivalent in the table below.

GRADE EQUIVALENT	
Raw Score	Grade Range
0-18	**3rd Grade and Below**
	Will not be able to read most low literacy materials; will need repeated oral instructions, materials composed primarily of illustrations, or audio or video tapes.
19-44	**4th to 6th Grade**
	Will need low literacy materials; may not be able to read prescription labels.
45-60	**7th to 8th Grade**
	Will struggle with most patient education materials; will not be offended by low literacy materials.
61-66	**High School**
	Will be able to read most patient education materials.

FIGURE 2-3 cont'd, Rapid Estimate of Adult Literacy in Medicine (REALM)©. (From Davis TL and others: Practical assessment of adult literacy in health care, *Health Educ Behav* 25:613-624, 1998.)

written materials provided for them by health professionals. Five percent of the adult population cannot read. Even the use of audiotaped instructions taxes the language and thinking skills of these persons. These patients may also have problems with basic clinician-patient communication (such as three times a day), lack the necessary vocabulary to ask pertinent questions,[13] and be unable to read prescriptions and follow medical recommendations. They have poorer knowledge of their diseases and worse clinical outcomes.[40]

Many individuals who are illiterate have normal or above normal intelligence. They will nearly always try to conceal their illiteracy and will use excuses such as not having time or having left their eyeglasses at home. They may be articulate and well dressed. Frequently, they "go along" and react positively even when they do not understand. However, illiterate persons cannot use reference documents or catalogs effectively, cannot follow instruction sheets, and cannot comprehend simple road maps.[22] In focus groups, low-literacy patients did not know what "orally" meant and were not sure whether medications for an ear infection should go in the mouth or in the ear.[35]

The consequences of this problem affect the patient and the caregiver responsible for the patient's well-being; the caregiver also faces the possibility of litigation initiated by a patient acting without knowledge that should have been provided. Thus, techniques known to be most effective should be used to teach these individuals.[15]

1. Eliminate everything that is extraneous.
2. Build to complexity when it is necessary; break content into components; and build with review, feedback, and questions.
3. Require patients to demonstrate what they have learned.
4. Give more rewards to those who are insecure in their ability to learn; they need more rewards than do others to accomplish small tasks.
5. To reduce the reading level and literacy demand, use a conversational style, active voice, short words, and short sentences.
6. Use visual aids, especially line drawings, with only one idea portrayed in each picture; use captions not longer than 10 words.
7. Clearly show correct behavior.
8. Organize material in the order patients will use it, and use words that are familiar to them.
9. Pretest all materials.
10. Use stories.

An example of a pamphlet for patients with limited literacy may be found in Figure 2-4. This is written at a lower reading level than the sixth grade level recommended for instructional materials (75% of adult Americans are able to read at this level).[15] Other teaching approaches such as demonstration, group activities, and discussions may be more effective with these populations.

An intervention for low literacy persons with diabetes incorporates many of the suggestions made above. Literacy was assessed by REALM. The intervention included 1:1 educational sessions and phone contact, focusing only on critical behaviors, decreasing complexity, using concrete examples, and limiting the number of topics in one session.[40]

Computers

Computers are used for instructional purposes such as drill and practice in problem solving with feedback until a skill is mastered, for games, and as simulators in which one learns how, for example, to adjust insulin level with a program that models the body's blood glucose and responses to insulin, diet, and exercise. A recently described diabetes management model using the Internet allowed immediate exchange of information between physicians and patients and showed a marked decrease in hemoglobin A_{1c} levels after 12 weeks in comparison with usual care.[31] On the basis of an on-line assessment of what the patient understands, computers can provide highly individualized self-paced learning and can document the learning process. They can be used to elicit information from patients that can help tailor patient education and discharge planning. They can include photographs and videos and narrated sound tracks for those with limited reading skills.

ComputerLink is a computer network that has been used to provide information and decision-support functions for caregivers of persons with Alzheimer's disease. A recent study[6] showed that this system enhanced the caregivers' confidence

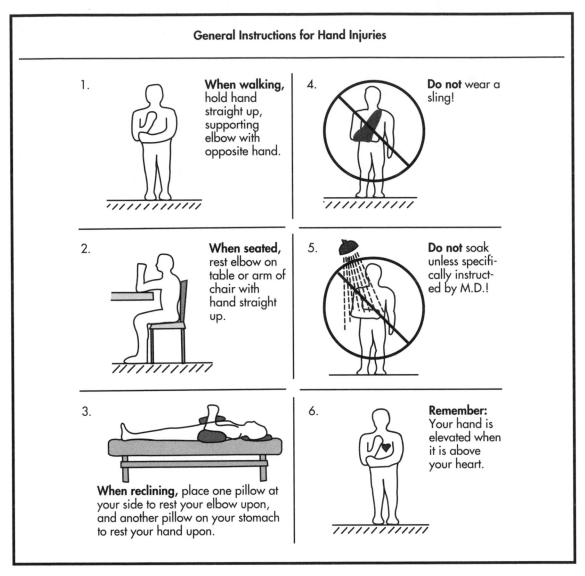

FIGURE 2-4 General instructions for hand injuries. (From Dooley AR: A collaborative model for creating patient education resources, *Am J Health Behav* 20:15-19, 1996.)

and decreased their sense of isolation, which is especially important in that other services are inaccessible because they require leaving home.[7]

A behavioral treatment program for obesity uses an interactive microcomputer small enough to be carried by subjects during their normal daily routines. Learners make self-reports on consumption of food and exercise. If they forget to do so, they are reminded by the computer.

Computerized training (by CD-ROM) in breast self-examination with use of a breast model and computer-guided feedback on accuracy of lump detection yielded a higher sense of self-efficacy among users of a federally qualified health center than did use of a pamphlet. For many women, self-efficacy translates into a range of operational details such as understanding the breast anatomy, knowing what lumps feel like, and understanding how much pressure to apply in an examination. The CD-ROM showed moving video testimonies regarding the value of breast self-examination, an interactive program that prompts the user to explore the model to find lumps (a lump identified in the model can be located on the computer screen with a mouse click) and what to do if a lump is found. Skill and confidence in breast self-examination is especially important for women who cannot afford regular access to primary health care services and therefore may have to be more reliant for monitoring their own health status.[39]

Visual Materials

In teaching about actual physical objects, it is often preferable to use the real thing. Nothing but a baby can act like a baby during a bath. However, models are useful when three dimensions must be retained but (1) the real thing is too small, large, complicated, or expensive; (2) the real thing is unavailable; (3) the desired view cannot be exposed; or (4) the object cannot be manipulated. For example, for demonstrating the birth of a baby, a doll may be advanced through an actual-size model of the bony structure of the pelvis. Many times, anatomy and physiology cannot be adequately visualized with the use of a real person because other tissues are in the way or a body part, such as the eye, is too small and complex. A dummy can be useful for showing the position of a tracheostomy and how to remove and reinsert parts of the tube. It can also be used for practicing general movements with the suction tube. The dummy is clearly limited because it lacks functioning muscles and secretions. Some teachers would insist that it is better to start the learner working with a real tracheostoma. However, if a patient with one is not available, or if the available patient's tracheostoma is difficult to care for, early practice on a model may be helpful. Models in the form of dummies are used to teach resuscitation techniques because a person whose heart or breathing has stopped is not usually available. Or a model the size of a

3-year-old child, with a bladder, can be used to teach clean intermittent catheterization to children to lessen their incontinence to an acceptable level.[10]

Thus models may be used because they can teach better than real objects can or because they are more practical to use. At times they are absolutely essential. However, models are frequently expensive and may not be readily available in many places where patients are being taught.

The research literature on pictorial learning is sparse in comparison with that on verbal learning. The theory of how people learn from pictures is not completely developed. Pictorial learning is superior to verbal learning for recognition and recall. For example, pictographs (pictures that represent ideas and assist in their recall) attain meaning when they are explained and remind the person of the associated idea. A drawing of a toothbrush, teeth, three vertical lines, and the sun and moon are a reminder to brush teeth three times a day.[25] However, when the subject matter is abstract, it is difficult to communicate with pictures. Media used to convey pictures always distort the various visual dimensions—resolution, color fidelity, and size—to some degree. For example, paintings may eliminate or exaggerate various parts of an object. These distortions may or may not be important to a particular learning task.

Photographs and drawings lack the third dimension but are readily available or can be produced by the teacher. The third dimension is not imperative when the teacher is showing familiar objects or those in which shape and space are not the primary considerations. Examples that fall into these categories and are frequently not available include an infected finger or an abnormal stool in infants. However, the learner must be aware that odor can be important in recognizing abnormal stool. In both of these examples, photographs would be more desirable than diagrams because they more accurately portray the details of the real item.

Drawings are particularly pertinent for removing superfluous detail present in real objects. During an explanation to a patient about diverticulitis, visualization is obviously desirable. Whereas a photograph shows details of the tissue that the patient does not need to know, a simple line drawing can communicate the concept of a pouch in the intestinal wall. In other instances, drawings in the form of cartoons are used to create interest in a topic. Figure 2-4 presents instructions for hand injuries graphically enhanced and illustrated to improve patient understanding.[16]

Pictures may be presented in many ways, depending on the size of the audience and equipment available. For a single individual, visuals on paper $8^1/_2$ by 11 inches can be used. For small groups, posters can be prepared. Drawings can be made with crayons or felt-tipped pens on flip charts (pads of paper approximately 32 by 26 inches) supported on an easel or chair back. Cutouts can be attached by magnets or flannel to metal or flannel boards. Drawings can be done on the chalkboard. A wide range of visual materials can be shown by computer.

Videos can be used as "triggers," providing an instructional stimulus that can be followed by discussion groups. In addition, the teacher can use images of the patient's own cardiac catheterization to teach both the patient and the family about the extent or the absence of cardiac problems. This approach eliminates generic information in other educational tools that may not be immediately useful to a particular patient.

An excellent example of a culturally relevant video was made to increase awareness about breast cancer and mammography screening among low-literacy Latinas in the precontemplation stage of behavior change.[6] According to the Health Belief Model, Latinas' perceived barriers included the belief that cancer is fatal, embarrassment, and limited English ability. Perceived severity of breast cancer is high, but their own perceived susceptibility to the illness is very low. The 8-minute video was created in an entertainment-education soap opera format, incorporating cultural values such as family as central, social interdependence, preference for personal interactions, deference and respect for authority figures, and a view of health as holistic. This group preferred storytelling from ethnic characters presenting information in an entertaining manner in a group setting. Characters were positive role models, including those who initially either opposed or were unaware of the educational objectives but then reversed their position, moving to contemplation and action stages. Along with the video, a flip chart contains follow-up questions for the group

Decision Aids. Patients face an increasing number of complex choices regarding prevention, diagnosis, and treatment, making it important that they understand the probabilities of various outcomes and their relative preferences for each option. Decision aids are teaching tools that also focus on assisting patients to make choices as part of the move to informed choice and shared decision making with providers, particularly where outcomes are uncertain or options have different benefit-risk profiles. Some have vicarious experiences or exercises designed to help clarify patients' values regarding the decision at hand. They are adjuncts to rather than substitutes for patient-physician interaction. Forms can be written or oral, decision boards, linear videotapes, and interactional computer-driven multimedia programs. Desired outcomes are increased knowledge, a decision consistent with the patient's values, satisfaction with it, and acted on.[4] Decision aids have the greatest effect on the choices of those who are undecided at baseline.[38]

Two examples of decision aids show how they are different from more traditional forms of patient education. Man-Son-Hing and others[33] describe development of a decision aid for patients with atrial fibrillation who are considering antithrombotic therapy. These patients are five times more likely to have a stroke compared with those without atrial fibrillation. To prevent stroke, warfarin is more efficacious than is aspirin but has a greater number of adverse effects and is more inconvenient to use. This decision aid was developed in the form of an audio-booklet, presenting the probabilities of stroke and major hemorrhage by use of facial icons (Figure 2-5). On a worksheet patients clarified their values, recorded questions or comments, and indicated their preferences (Figure 2-6). Patients using this aid were more likely than were control patients to make a definitive choice regarding anti-thrombotic therapy, were more knowledgeable, and were slightly less likely to choose to take warfarin.

Choices	Stroke and Bleeding Risk	Points to Consider

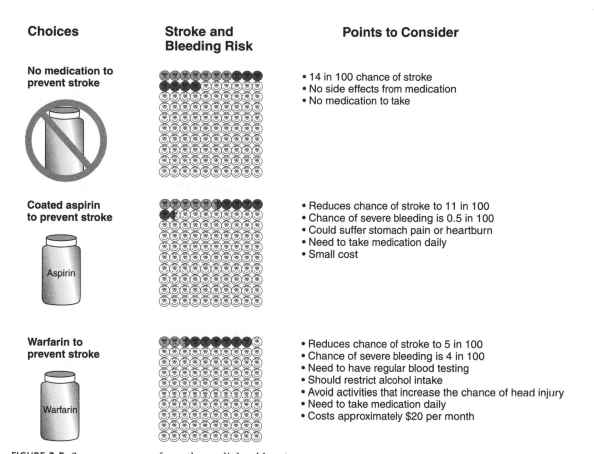

No medication to prevent stroke

- 14 in 100 chance of stroke
- No side effects from medication
- No medication to take

Coated aspirin to prevent stroke

Aspirin

- Reduces chance of stroke to 11 in 100
- Chance of severe bleeding is 0.5 in 100
- Could suffer stomach pain or heartburn
- Need to take medication daily
- Small cost

Warfarin to prevent stroke

Warfarin

- Reduces chance of stroke to 5 in 100
- Chance of severe bleeding is 4 in 100
- Need to have regular blood testing
- Should restrict alcohol intake
- Avoid activities that increase the chance of head injury
- Need to take medication daily
- Costs approximately $20 per month

FIGURE 2-5 Summary pages from the audiobooklet. (From Man-Son-Hing M and others: Development of a decision aid for patients with atrial fibrillation who are considering antithrombotic therapy, *J Gen Intern Med* 15:723-730, 2000.)

Green and others[21] describe an interactive, multimedia, computer-based decision aid to educate individuals and help facilitate informed decision making about genetic testing for breast cancer susceptibility among women with family or personal histories of breast cancer. In comparison with standard genetic counseling, women using the aid were more knowledgeable and those using counseling more accurate in their risk perceptions (in this case, the decision aid did not provide individualized risk assessments). For women at high risk or those in need of additional psychosocial support, the computer is best used as a supplement to rather than as a replacement for genetic counseling. For those at low risk, the decision aid has the potential to stand alone, important because of the extreme shortage of genetic counselors.

Screening, Preparing, and Testing Teaching Materials

All materials must be viewed and evaluated before they are used for teaching. Previewing is necessary to identify material that the teacher believes is incorrect or is contradictory to other sources being used. It may be necessary to reject an audiovisual aid because it is beyond the level of the learners' understanding or because the aid may be peripheral to the objectives. Materials must also be culturally relevant.

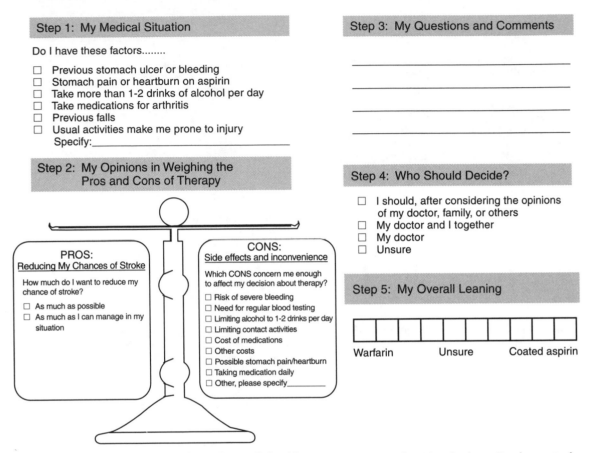

FIGURE 2-6 Personal worksheet from the audiobooklet. (From Man-Son-Hing M and others: Development of a decision aid for patients with atrial fibrillation who are considering antithrombotic therapy, *J Gen Intern Med* 15:723-730, 2000.)

After preview, an instructional material or product should undergo two steps to improve its effectiveness as a teaching tool.

1. Product verification. Arrange a tryout of the materials under conditions approximating those in which the finally developed product will be used, using a pretest measure on each instructional objective; record time spent on program components, teacher-learner behavior, and other relevant measures of student use of the material; use a postassessment measure; and release the materials for general use if performance is high on all objectives.

2. Product revision. Identify the objectives not well met; from data gathered in the verifica-

tion step, propose revisions; test the revised version.

Learner data are most important in judging learnability. A more complete testing program should be used when there is no precedent for either the content or teaching method, when learning materials are more complex and expensive, when the materials seek to change attitudes rather than to increase knowledge, when materials are designed for long-term rather than short-term use, and when the target audience is large. This involves repetitive tryouts with individuals to identify major errors, repetitive tryouts with small groups, and a field test when the materials are well developed.

Sets of criteria for quality instructional materials, developed by two different authors, may be found in Box 2-7.[5] The criteria by Doak, Doak, and Root are scored into the Suitability Assessment of Materials and particularly incorporate literacy-relevant factors (Figure 2-7).[15]

Planning and Implementing Instruction

All items necessary for constructing a teaching plan have been introduced. Evaluation, which is also part of the plan, is discussed thoroughly in Chapter 3. Because the purpose of a teaching plan is to force the teacher to examine the relationships among learner receptivity, objectives, content,

Box 2-7	*Domain of Instructional Design Principles Survey*

1. Drawings/illustrations represent racial and ethnic groups.
2. The learning objectives are made clear to the target group.
3. The size of the PEM is one that is easily handled by the target group (5×8 inches is easy to handle; 8×10 inches is easy to file).
4. The learning objectives cover the main points to be learned from the PEM.
5. The learning objectives for the PEM and the procedures for accomplishing them are distinguishable.
6. The relevance of the educational content to the target group is clearly stated.
7. Only the most essential information is presented, using not more than 3 to 4 main points (i.e., what, where, when, and how).
8. Sentence parts are kept in logical order.
9. Titles and subtitles are clear and informative.
10. There is sufficient contrast between the ink and the paper to make reading easy.
11. Drawings/illustrations are labeled clearly.
12. The use of double (or multiple) negatives in sentences is avoided.
13. The content is presented in an unbiased manner that respects free choice on the part of the target group.
14. The content is presented in a way that relates and integrates the new information to what is already known and understood by the target group.
15. Mnemonic devices are used as retrieval cues for important information (e.g., ABC = *Airway, Breaths,* and *Compressions* for cardiopulmonary resuscitation).
16. The material builds from the familiar to the unfamiliar.
17. The educational content is appropriate to community standards.
18. The focus of the PEM is on how to accomplish the learning task.
19. The educational content is written in a style that is patient centered and specific.
20. The content includes descriptions of physical sensations that the target group is likely to experience during diagnostic and therapeutic procedures.
21. The vocabulary of the PEM comprises words commonly used by the target group.
22. Important ideas and points of content are repeated as reinforcement throughout the PEM.
23. Important information is organized as lists or categories.
24. The information most important to the target group is presented first.
25. One idea per paragraph is presented.
26. Short, simple sentences are used to convey one idea at a time.
27. Terms are used in a consistent manner throughout the PEM.
28. Supplemental information is separated from the main points and is provided as an appendix or other special section.
29. The PEM includes a space for patient-generated questions.

Box 2-7	*Domain of Instructional Design Principles Survey—cont'd*

30. A listing of resources that provide additional information about the topic is included in the PEM.
31. Necessary health terms are defined.
32. Topic headings and advance organizers (eg, topic outlines, introductory summaries) are used.
33. The content is presented in concrete terms rather than as abstract concepts and ideas.
34. The first sentence of each paragraph is the topic sentence.
35. Specific, precise instructions are given if the target group is expected to carry out some self-care activity.
36. The title of the PEM is short and conveys the meaning of the material.
37. Drawings/illustrations are recognizable to the target group with or without explanatory text.
38. A table of contents is provided for PEMs that are lengthy.
39. The table of contents is designed to match the readers' questions.
40. The PEM includes a space for patient-generated questions.
41. The content focuses on what the target group should do as well as what they need to know.
42. Drawings/illustrations accurately convey the content to improve understanding of the material.
43. Opportunities are provided in the text for the target group to use the new concepts just presented.
44. The main ideas of the PEM are divided into meaningful content units.
45. Drawings/illustrations present only essential content relevant to the educational purpose.
46. Specialized vocabulary lists are developed and placed at the front of the PEM for easy reader access.
47. Ideas are expressed using one- to two-syllable words as much as possible.
48. Drawings/illustrations are placed next to the text to which they refer.
49. The font or print size is easily read by the target group.
50. The second person, *you*, is used instead of the third person except in situations where the content may be emotionally charged (e.g., cancer or AIDS information).
51. The type style is easy to read.
52. The paper used in the PEM is of a nonglare (uncoated) type for ease of reading.
53. The lines of drawings/illustrations are heavy enough to be seen by the target group.
54. Questions are posed throughout the PEM as a means of engaging the reader in the content and highlighting the main points.
55. Contractions are used to make the text more personal (e.g., *you'll* instead of *you will*).
56. A positive writing style is used.
57. The content is verified as accurate by persons experienced in the content area.
58. Consideration is given to eye span of the text (e.g., 50-70 characters per line is most comfortable for reading).
59. The tone of the PEM is personal and nonthreatening.
60. Equal consideration to gender is given in the use of pronouns.
61. The content is respectful of the customs and traditions of the target group.
62. The writing style is one that engages the reader and stimulates active participation.
63. The PEM is written at a readability level that is appropriate to the target group (e.g., material intended for the general public should be written at the sixth- to eight-grade level).
64. The leading (space between each line of type) used facilitates reading (10-point type requires 2 points of leading; 11-point type requires 3 points, very small type requires more leading to make text less dense and more readable).
65. Color is used as a cuing agent to highlight materials and promote learning.
66. Drawings/illustrations represent gender equally where content is appropriate to both sexes.
67. Each drawing/illustration conveys a single idea or concept.

Box 2-7	*Domain of Instructional Design Principles Survey—cont'd*

68. The purpose of the PEM is made clear to the target group of learners.
69. PEMs intended for long-term use are constructed of materials that will withstand handling and use.
70. The material moves from simpler to more complex content in a manner that is organized and logical.
71. The examples used in the PEM contain the central characteristics of the ideas and concepts under discussion.
72. Examples are used to bridge the gap between what the target group already knows and the content to be taught.
73. Both upper and lower case letters are used for ease of reading.
74. The information load of the material (amount of information and novelty/obscurity of information) is appropriate to the target group.
75. The most important information is highlighted in bold print.
76. The spacing and layout of text and drawings/illustrations are attractive and pleasing to the eye.
77. The lines of the text are justified for ease of reading.
78. The learning objectives and educational content of the PEM relate to one another.
79. The active voice is used.
80. The learning objectives of the PEM are related to the intended outcome.
81. Arabic numbers are used to facilitate ease of reading when numbers are included in the educational content.
82. The cover of the PEM is attractive and eye catching.
83. The PEM has esthetic appeal.
84. The first lines of paragraphs are indented for ease of reading.
85. The margins surrounding the text are wide enough to provide ease of reading and space for note taking by the target group.
86. The educational content is current.
87. Accurate and coherent summaries/synopsis of the message being delivered are included throughout the PEM.
88. Numbers are written as numbers rather than as text.
89. The ideas being presented in the PEM are logically related and present a coherent structure for the information being conveyed.
90. The colors used in the PEM should be in keeping with the mood of the topic.

PEM, Patient education material.
From Bernier MJ: Establishing the psychometric properties of a scale for evaluating quality in printed education materials, *Patient Educ Couns* 29:293-299, 1996.

teaching methods, tools, and evaluation, a plan should be written.

Teaching plans can be written in many formats. The major criterion for judging a format is whether it clearly states the various elements of the teaching process. Are the relationships among assessment-readiness, objectives, teaching actions, and content and evaluation clear? Is the format easy to follow in the urgent atmosphere of teaching in a busy clinical situation? When teaching and learning are a major intervention, it is usual to construct a separate teaching plan, possibly one that can be incorporated into the general nursing care plan. An example appears in Figure 2-8. Increasingly, teaching is being incorporated into clinical pathways. Figure 2-9 shows

2 points for superior rating
1 point for adequate rating
0 points for not suitable rating
N/A if the factor does not apply to this material

FACTOR TO BE RATED	SCORE	COMMENTS

1. CONTENT

(a) Purpose is evident
(b) Content about behaviors
(c) Scope is limited
(d) Summary or review included

2. LITERACY DEMAND

(a) Reading grade level
(b) Writing style, active voice
(c) Vocabulary uses common words
(d) Context is given first
(e) Learning aids via "road signs"

3. GRAPHICS

(a) Cover graphic shows purpose
(b) Type of graphics
(c) Relevance of illustrations
(d) List, tables, etc., explained
(e) Captions used for graphics

4. LAYOUT AND TYPOGRAPHY

(a) Layout factors
(b) Typography
(c) Subheads ("chunking") used

5. LEARNING STIMULATION, MOTIVATION

(a) Interaction used
(b) Behaviors are modeled and specific
(c) Motivation—self-efficacy

6. CULTURAL APPROPRIATENESS

(a) Match in logic, language, experience
(b) Cultural image and examples

Total SAM score: _____

Total possible score: _____ Percent score: _____ %

FIGURE 2-7 SAM (Suitability Assessment of Materials) scoring sheet. (From Doak CC, Doak LG, Root JH: *Teaching patients with low literacy skills*, ed 2, Philadelphia, 1996, Lippincott.)

SAMPLE STANDARD TEACHING PLAN
Mutliple Sclerosis

Patient Learning Objectives	Content		Education Mode	Modifications/Comments	Objectives Met (Date/Initials)
Patient will define the remission/ exacerbation aspects of the disease process.	Infection, trauma, immunization, delivery after pregnancy, stress, climactic changes How remission/exacerbation is experienced		E D		
Patient will demonstrate how to use various community resources.	Local and national multiple sclerosis society chapters Public health nurse Visiting Nurse Association Community support groups Social workers, therapists Vocational rehabilitation agencies Home health agencies Extended and skilled care facilities Financial counseling		E P V RP		
Patient will specify the safety precautions associated with symptoms.	Decreased sensation Visual disturbances Motor deficits	Safety precautions	E R P		
Patient will take medications correctly and will recognize expected effects and side effects and interactions with over-the-counter medicines associated with each medication.	Corticosteroids Immunomodulators Cholinergics Anticholinergics Muscle relaxants	How to take— recognizing expected effects and side effects	E R RP		
Patient will perform exercises to promote muscle strength and mobility.	Measures for preventing contractures and skin breakdown Transfer techniques and proper body mechanics Use of assistive devices and other measures to minimize neurological deficits		E R V M		
Patient will diagnose and self-manage constipation, urinary retention, or urinary tract infection (UTI), including proper self-catheterization technique or care of indwelling urinary catheters.	Constipation Urinary retention UTI	How to diagnosis and self-manage	E R		

FIGURE **2-8** Sample standard teaching plan.

an example of a basic pathway. This format can be modified for any diagnosis and also used as a documentation tool.[18]

Availability of good standards of care, teaching tools, and forms for recording teaching is essential to ensure that teaching is actually being delivered to patients.

In purposeful, planned teaching, the caregiver carries out the plan, which can be used as a guide unless feedback from the patient indicates clearly that it is inappropriate or ineffective. If this happens, the planning process must be repeated, and new data must be added. Experienced teachers can do that on the spot and move ahead. Others will need to stop the teaching session and, if possible, replan and reimplement.

Staff training is also important to implement programs. Traditional methods of teaching health professionals how to teach often focus only on the theoretical aspects of the teaching-learning

Patient Learning Objectives	Content	Education Mode	Modifications/Comments	Objectives Met (Date/Initials)
Patient will identify indications of upper respiratory infection and implementation of measures that help prevent regurgitation, aspiration, and respiratory infection.	Cough, increased nasal and respiratory secretions, inability to tolerate breathing of cold air, temperature 100.4° F (38° C), dysphagia How to manage these effects	E V		
Patient will alter diet as necessary.	A nutritious, well-balanced diet Soft food for patients with chewing difficulties High-fiber diet for patients experiencing constipation	E V P M		
Patient will relate the importance of follow-up care to achieve desired outcomes.	Visits to physician Visits to physical therapist Visits to occupational therapists Speech, sexual, or psychological counseling	E P V		

Resource Box (list available patient resources here):

Education Mode Key	Signature	Initial
P = Pamphlet B = Book R = Reciprocal demonstration D = Dialogue E = Explication V = Video RP= Role playing M = Modeling		

FIGURE 2-8 cont'd, Sample standard teaching plan.

process. Frequently, little help is offered to transfer this information into the practice setting. One approach involves apprenticing novice teachers to master teachers, allowing them to observe and participate and gradually do the teaching on their own with feedback from the master teacher. Videotaping teaching interactions provides an opportunity for self-evaluation and critique from a master teacher.

SUMMARY

Educational objectives are based on assessment of a patient's readiness and need to learn; they are the framework for the instructional plan. Instructional forms and teaching materials are identified or constructed to provide the learning conditions necessary for meeting the objectives. Teaching plans put these elements together and guide implementation.

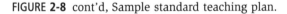

Study Questions

1. A study of patients with lacerations who were treated in an emergency department found that those whose discharge instructional materials contained illustrations were 1.5 times more likely to choose correct responses than were those whose instructions did not contain illustrations.[2] Does this finding surprise you?

BASIC CLINICAL PATHWAY

Patient name _____Admit _____
Primary diagnosis _____

Standard of care	Number of visits	Outcome	Initials
Physical and mental assessment Vital signs and blood pressure Mental and physical status Response to medications	Every visit	Temperature, pulse and blood pressure are within acceptable limits. Medication is producing desired effects.	

Educational assessment
Disease pathophysiology
  Definition
  Etiology
  Process/progression
  Causes of exacerbation
  Complications
	1-3	Patient/family comprehends information on disease pathophysiology.	

Medication teaching
  Use of drug
  Side effects
  Adverse reactions
	1-3	Patient/family is able to verbalize understanding of medications.	

Treatments/procedures	1-3	Patient is able to verbalize understanding of reason for treatment and able to perform treatment independently.	

Safety-related issues
  Emergency measures
  Universal precautions
  Safety in the home
	1
	1-2
	1-2
		Patient is able to access emergency care.
		Patient is able to protect self from safety or infection control related problems.	

Discharge planning Ongoing care needed for patient resource help	1-2	Patient/family understands discharge instructions. Patient verbalizes understanding for follow-up visits with physician.	

Quality management
Is pathway being followed?

Date ____Yes ____No ____   Date ____Yes ____No ____
Date ____Yes ____No ____   Date ____Yes ____No ____

If pathway is not followed, what is the variance and action plan?

Date _____Variance _____
Action plan _____
Date _____Variance _____
Action plan _____

FIGURE 2-9 Basic clinical pathway. (From Freeman SR, Chambers KA: Home health care: clinical pathways and quality integration, *Nurs Manag* 28:45-48, 1999.)

2. A mother comments to you, "My baby has clumsy fingers." You determine that the child's growth and development are normal for his/her age but that the child could profit from environmental stimulation to develop eye-hand coordination and prehension. What kinds of general teaching approaches might be used?

REFERENCES

1. Aldridge MD: Writing and designing readable patient education materials, *Nephrol Nurs J* 31:373-377, 2004.

2. Austin PE and others: Discharge instructions: do illustrations help our patients understand them? *Ann Emerg Med* 25:317-320, 1995.

3. Baker DW, Parker RM, Williams MV, Clark WS: Health literacy and the risk of hospital admission, *J Gen Intern Med* 13;791-798, 1998.

4. Barry MJ: Health decision aids to facilitate shared decision making in office practice, *Ann Intern Med* 136:127-135, 2002.

5. Bernier MJ: Establishing the psychometric properties of a scale for evaluating quality in printed education materials, *Patient Educ Couns* 29:283-299, 1996.

6. Borrayo EA: Where's Maria? A video to increase awareness about breast cancer and mammography screening among low-literacy Latinas, *Prev Med* 39:99-110, 2004.

7. Brennan PF, Moore SM, Smyth KA: The effects of a special computer network on caregivers of persons with Alzheimer's disease, *Nurs Res* 44:166-172, 1995.

8. Bulechek GM and others: Nursing interventions used in practice, *Am J Nurs* 94:59-64, 1994.

9. Buxton T: Effective ways to improve health education materials, *J Health Educ* 30:47-50, 61, 1999.

10. Cobussen-Boekhorst JGL, Van Der Weide M, Feitz WFJ, De Gier RPE: Using an instructional model to teach clean intermittent catheterization to children, *BJU Internat* 85:551-553, 2000.

11. Colagiuri R, Colagiuri S, Naidu V: Can patients set their own educational priorities? *Diabetes Res Clin Pract* 30:131-136, 1995.

12. Crowe L, Billingsley JI: The rowdy reactors: maintaining a support group for teenagers with diabetes, *Diabetes Educ* 16:39-43, 1990.

13. Davis TL and others: Practical assessment of adult literacy in health care, *Health Educ Behav* 25: 613-624, 1998.

14. DeBasio N, Rodenhausen N: The group experience: meeting the psychological needs of patients with ventricular tachycardia, *Heart Lung* 13:597-602, 1984.

15. Doak CC, Doak LG, Root JH: *Teaching patients with low literacy skills*, ed 2, Philadelphia, 1996, Lippincott.

16. Dooley AR: A collaborative model for creating patient education resources, *Am J Health Behav* 20:15-19, 1996.

17. Freda MC, Damus K, Merkatz IR: Evaluation of the readability of ACOG patient education pamphlets, *Obstet Gynecol* 93:771-774, 1999.

18. Freeman SR, Chambers KA: Home health care; clinical pathways and quality integration, *Nurs Manag* 28:45-48, 1999.

19. Gagliano ME: A literature review on the efficacy of video in patient education, *J Med Educ* 63:785-792, 1988.

20. Graber MA, Roller CM, Kaeble B: Readability levels of patient education material on the World Wide Web, *J Fam Pract* 48:58-61, 1999.

21. Green MJ and others: Effect of a computer-based decision aid on knowledge, perceptions and intentions about genetic testing for breast cancer susceptibility, *JAMA* 292:442-452, 2004.

22. Greene VL, Monahan DJ: The effect of a professional guided caregiver support and education group on institutionalization of care receivers, *Gerontologist* 27:716-721, 1987.

23. Gronlund NE: *Writing instructional objectives for teaching and assessment*, 7th ed, Upper Saddle River, NJ, 2004, Pearson Merrill Prentice-Hall.

24. Holt CI, Kyles A, Wiebagen T, Casey C: Development of a spiritually based breast cancer educational booklet for African-American women, *Cancer Control* 10(5 Suppl): 37-44, 2003.

25. Houts PS and others: Using pictographs to enhance recall and spoken medical instructions, *Patient Educ Couns* 35:83-88, 1998.

26. Iowa Intervention Project: Validation and coding of the NIC taxonomy structure, *Image* 27:43-49, 1995.

27. Jacobs MK, Goodman G: Psychology and self-help groups, *Am Psychol* 44:536-545, 1989.

28. Janz NK, Becher MH, Hartman PE: Contingency contracting to enhance patient compliance: a review, *Patient Educ Couns* 5:164-178, 1984.

29. Kozma RB: Learning with media, *Rev Educ Res* 61: 179-211, 1991.

30. Kulik JA, Mahler HIM: Effects of preoperative roommate assignments on preoperative anxiety and recovery from coronary bypass surgery, *Health Psychol* 6:525-543, 1987.

31. Kwon HS and others: Establishment of blood glucose monitoring system using the internet. *Diabetes Care* 27:478-483, 2004.

32. Lasater L, Mehler PS: The illiterate patient: screening and management, *Hosp Pract* 33:163-170, 1998.

33. Man-Son-Hing M and others: Development of a decision aid for patients with atrial fibrillation who are considering antithrombotic therapy. *J Gen Intern Med* 15:723-730, 2000.

34. Massett HA: Appropriateness of Hispanic print materials: a content analysis, *Health Educ Res* 11:231-242, 1996.

35. Mayeaux EJ and others: Improving patient education for patients with low literacy skills, *Am Fam Physician* 53:205-211, 1996.

36. Myers RE, Shepard-White F: Evaluation of adequacy of reading level and readability of psychotropic medication handouts, *J Am Psychiatr Nurses Assoc* 10:55-59, 2004.

37. Nurss JR, Parker RM, Williams MV, Baker DW: *Test of functional health literacy in adults*, Atlanta, 1995, Center for the Study of Adult Literacy, Georgia State University.

38. O'Connor AM and others: Decision aids for patients considering options affecting cancer outcomes: evidence of efficacy and policy implications, *Monogr Natl Cancer Inst* 25:67-80, 1999.

39. Reis J, Trockel M, King T, Remmert D: Computerized training in breast self-examination, *Cancer Nurs* 27:162-168, 2004.

40. Rothman RL and others: Influence of patient literacy on the effectiveness of a primary care-based diabetes disease management program, *JAMA* 292:1711-1716, 2004.

41. Walling AM, Maliski S, Bogorad A, Litwin MS: Assessment of content completeness and accuracy of prostate cancer patient education materials. *Patient Educ Coun* 54:337-343, 2004.

3

Evaluation in Patient Education

Evaluation determines the worth of something by judging it against a standard, usually stated as a learning objective and defined by a field of practice or study. Evaluation can serve several purposes. It can direct and motivate learning because it provides evidence about patients' accomplishments or skills that they need to develop. Evaluation can also be used to judge whether someone ought to be selected or certified for having met a particular level of expertise. Patient education generally has not been used to provide a formal certification; however, evaluative judgments about learning commonly provide the basis for allowing a patient to progress to another setting, such as home. Evaluation also reinforces correct behavior on the part of learners and helps teachers determine the adequacy of their teaching. In each situation it is important to think through the purpose of the evaluation first.

Once the standard is clear, the next step is to assign evaluative tasks to the learners. Ambiguous tasks produce faulty evidence and lead to faulty conclusions concerning how much the patient has learned. As a result, the learner is confused.

Evidence is compared with criteria or standards of adequate performance, and a judgment of adequacy or inadequacy is made. The teaching that follows a judgment of inadequate learning can correct errors in the patient's performance, present correct behavior, and explain the errors and correct behavior, as well as improve teaching.

Evaluating programs of patient education is also necessary for teaching groups of patients over a period of time. Program evaluation provides direction for improvement of learning in individual patients and leads to judgments about how to improve the program.

In the current state of patient education practice, purposive evaluation is not routinely carried out; indeed, learning goals (which are the basis for evaluation) are frequently not clearly stated. In addition, the most useful outcomes from patient education (problem solving in real-life situations) are frequently not used. For example, the most common outcome measure from diabetes education is patient knowledge about glycosylated hemoglobin. Knowledge appears to be necessary but not sufficient to produce adequate patient self-management skills and functioning; therefore, measures of knowledge may more properly be thought of as process measures on the way to other outcomes.[4] Hemoglobin A_{1C} is a physiologic measure of blood sugar levels over a 3-month time period; it is affected by many things other than patient skills and knowledge.

Clinical success has traditionally been appraised in terms of mortality and physiologic measures such as blood pressure, laboratory tests, x-ray study findings, and definable clinical events. Increasingly, patients' perceptions of symptoms, their ability to function in everyday life, their satisfaction with care, and their ability to make health care decisions are seen as important and predictive of future use of health care services.[1] A taxonomy of nurse-sensitive outcomes of patient care more closely related to outcomes of patient education is available.[8] Outcomes relevant to patient education include anxiety control, caregiver performance, perceived ability to perform, and participation in health care behaviors. Lorig and others[10] define a set of outcomes from self-management education for chronic diseases, which include self-management behaviors (e.g., exercise, cognitive symptom management, mental stress management, use of community services, and communication with providers) and self-efficacy for self-management behaviors for disease management in general and to achieve outcomes such as management of depression and symptoms and health states such as disability and social role limitations.

Although many formally developed measurement tools are available, they are not routinely used in clinical practice. Those with appropriate psychometric characteristics should be used—this is the only way clinical practice judgments will become more objective and reliable. Increasingly, disease management programs form the organizational structure in which outcomes are assessed and care processes improved. Review of a hospitalization may show that it was precipitated by lack of self-management skills. In reviewing the case, the nurse case manager determines that self-management education is needed. After the education is accomplished, the patient's recovery is tracked to see whether the education was effective.

OBTAINING MEASURES OF BEHAVIOR

All measurement involves observation of behavior. Such observation is more or less direct. Observations are more direct if the method of measurement involves viewing actual behavior as it occurs in natural settings and having access to its intended meaning. They are less direct if the method of measurement involves the subject's response to substitute situations that may be largely verbal and require much inference of intended meaning. Each method contains certain weaknesses that can produce error in measurement.

Because one of the major purposes of measurement and evaluation activities is to predict how the individual will behave in the future, it is best to base this prediction on observation of actual behavior (direct measurement). What people say they will do and what they actually do may be different. People often respond in ways that are socially acceptable rather than reveal their real feelings. Direct observation of behavior when the individual is unaware of being observed is the best opportunity for accurate assessment.

Although indirect measurements contain error, they also possess advantages that can contribute greatly to accurate assessment. Natural behavior is often inaccessible because it occurs in private—in family interactions. Natural behavior might occur infrequently and in various places. For example, it might surface in response to emergencies that require resuscitation measures, such as insulin shock, diabetic coma, or ingestion of poisons by a child.

Natural behavior might also occur infrequently, that is, at times when the observer may not be present. The strategy behind most tests used in indirect measurement is to present the situation in such a way that the provider can elicit the desired behavior in a written, oral, or performance response to a mock situation. Test results for complex behaviors are more accurate if the learner responds to situations on videotape rather than responding to written test situations.

Thus far in this chapter several major sources of error in measurement have been identified. One source of error is the constant possibility that indirect measures may present a false picture of an individual's behavior. A second source of error lies in the complexity of behavior. An observer may be unable to identify the causes of a particular behavior or be unable to measure thought patterns and attitudes even by direct observation. A third source is the bias of human observers. Observers cannot attend to or record all stimuli. They tend to assign meanings according to their own views. A fourth source of error is sampling. It is often not feasible in terms of time and effort expended to observe an individual's or a group's behavior repeatedly to account for the variation in performance from day to day and from situation to situation. It is not possible to inventory all aspects of an individual's knowledge about a particular subject. Obtaining samples over a period of time and in general areas of subject matter decreases error to an acceptable level.

The degree of error allowable depends on the predictions and decisions made and on the precision of the best measuring tool available. The provider should be more concerned with the person who needs to know how to care for a child's tracheostomy at home than with the person who needs to know how to do prenatal exercises. In both cases, observing the learner engaged in the behavior would provide appropriate data for evaluation. However, for tracheostomy care the teacher should observe many times, measuring the learner's behavior against objective criteria agreed on by experts. To evaluate the learner's understanding, the caregiver can supplement the observation with oral or written questions, asking the learner what to do if the tube becomes dislodged or why suctioning is done a particular way. All methods of measurement are prone to particular errors. To arrive at a decision, the best information often can be gained by using a combination of methods.

Measurement involves obtaining a record of pertinent behavior. Not only is it difficult to record all that occurs, but also this mass of information is not useful. The guideline for the pertinence of recording behavior is the statement of objectives. If the statement has met all the specifications for preciseness and clarity outlined in Chapter 2, it is much easier to decide which information is useful to record. Envision the difference in trying to evaluate these two patient objectives: (1) to know injection sites and (2) to draw on his or her own skin five areas suitable for injection of insulin. It is difficult to identify and measure the content and behavior of objective number 1. Note that no time is stipulated in this objective. Tests limiting time are appropriate only if the learned behavior requires speed.

Rating Scales and Checklists

The most complete recording of behavior is obtained from videotape. This method offers the added advantage that it can be reviewed with the learner to offer feedback on performance. A videotape, however, does not provide access to the learner's thinking unless he or she verbalizes it while recording. By itself it does not summarize the kind of behavior seen or identify its meaning in relation to objectives. To fill this need, a rating scale that describes pertinent behavior in words (anchored) can be constructed.

To reduce error in measurement, these words must be precise so that misinterpretation is avoided. For example, the rating scale (Box 3-1) can be refined so that several teachers who are observing a learner's behavior can independently classify it at one of the three points with little variation. If the raters cannot agree, the wording probably needs to be clarified. After the scale is refined, individual caregivers can use it by themselves.

Of course, it is possible for an individual to display behavior from two different levels of functioning (see descriptions of behavior in Box 3-1). For example, the patient may contaminate the syringe and needle fairly often (lowest level) but be quite skilled at removing bubbles from the syringe and measuring accurately (highest level). Behaviors are usually at adjacent levels on the rating scale because certain skills involve comparable levels of coordination. The difference may be that the learner is careless about contaminating. Checks can be made beside individual statements at various levels of the description. This will ensure that the teacher does not lose information about the learner's performance by checking just one of the categories on the line.

Box 3-1	*Sample Rating Scale*

Subobjective: To obtain 1 ml of aqueous fluid for injection from a 2-ml vial with a 2-ml syringe, 22-gauge needle, using sterile technique.

Consistently uses contaminated syringe, needle, or top of vial. Cannot push needle through diaphragm. Is rarely aware of erring and if so usually does not know how to correct the error.	Occasionally contaminates. Can push needle through diaphragm. Has difficulty withdrawing all the fluid and obtaining accurate measurement (within 0.1 ml). Can usually diagnose errors while doing the procedure and correct them.	Rarely contaminates. Can obtain last few drops out of vial without damaging needle. Can measure within 0.1 ml even if bubbles are present. Can change needle or syringe if defective or contaminated. Corrects errors by self.

(Other scales can be developed for other subobjectives of the skill of giving an injection.)

Another alternative is construction of several scales for this particular subobjective, each dealing with one set of behaviors—maintenance of sterility, obtaining and measuring fluid, or handling errors. Space is usually left below each rating scale for comments. A well-developed scale includes all pertinent points and rarely requires extra written comments. The form is developed to preclude recording behavior by writing it out at great length.

Other factors in the construction of a rating scale, besides preciseness of the descriptions, contribute to its quality as a measuring instrument. One factor is the number of levels of achievement represented in the behavior descriptions. The sample rating scale given here uses three levels of achievement because it is difficult for an observer to discriminate among more than five levels of achievement. Four or five steps could have been used. Note that the kinds of behaviors described in the scale are those that are crucial to the success of the skill as described in the objective: asepsis, accuracy of measurement, and ability to perceive and correct errors. Concerns such as inserting the needle precisely through the center of the rubber stopper or the particular manner in which the syringe is grasped are not considered crucial. The following is an example of a checklist that could be used in lieu of the sample rating scale in Box 3-1.

☐ Scrubbed top of vial with disinfectant sponge
☐ Punctured rubber vial with needle without contaminating
☐ Withdrew all of fluid from vial
☐ Expelled excess air from syringe without losing fluid
☐ Measured fluid to within 0.1 ml of the correct dose

Boxes 3-2, 3-3, and 3-4 provide examples of rating scales—for breast self-examination, for patient satisfaction, and for rating the umbilical cord of a newborn. Do these instruments elicit critical data? Are the most important elements included? Are some more crucial than others? If so, should they be marked so that patients who cannot do critical steps are identified? Would two health care providers watching a patient perform this procedure give him or her the same number of points? Might it help to include further descriptors of correct performance for each step?

Oral Questioning

Oral questioning is a flexible form of measurement often used in combination with techniques such as observation. It attempts to reach those behaviors that cannot be easily observed. For example, a caregiver may ask patients questions to determine whether they understand the basis for their actions in performing a psychomotor

---

Box 3-2   *Breast Self-Examination Proficiency Rating Instrument*

Inspection	**Palpation**
Arms at sides	Hand behind head
Arms over head	Begins examination at 12 o'clock position
Hands on hips	Examines all parts of breast
Leaning forward:	Closely examines upper outer quadrant
Looks for symmetry, size, shape	Uses circular motion for each palpation
Looks for puckering, dimpling	Uses pads of fingers
Examines skin for color, texture, lesions	Presses firmly and deeply
Inspection Total	Squeezes nipple
	Inspects axilla
	Palpation Total
	Total

From Wood RY: Reliability and validity of a breast self examination proficiency rating instrument, *Eval Health Prof* 17:418-435, 1994.

Box 3-3   *Satisfaction with Decision Instrument*

You have been considering whether to consult your health care provider about hormone replacement therapy. Answer the following questions about your decision. Please indicate to what extent each statement is true for you AT THIS TIME.

  Use the following scale to answer the questions.
1 = strongly disagree
2 = disagree
3 = neither agree nor disagree
4 = agree
5 = strongly agree

1. I am satisfied that I am adequately informed about the issues important to my decision.
2. The decision I made was the best decision possible for me personally.
3. I am satisfied that my decision was consistent with my personal values.
4. I expect to successfully carry out (or continue to carry out) the decision I made.
5. I am satisfied that this was my decision to make.
6. I am satisfied with my decision.

From Holmes-Rovner M and others: Patient satisfaction with health care decisions, *Med Decis Making* 16:58-64, 1996.

---

skill. Oral questioning also allows construction of hypothetical situations that are not present in the actual teaching environment. Examples of these practices include asking a man learning to irrigate his colostomy why he is preparing the equipment as he is or asking a mother what she would do if her baby turned blue, which may include a demonstration of resuscitation techniques.

The method of oral questioning can be expensive in terms of the time it takes, particularly if it is done in a one-to-one teacher-learner relationship. The strength of oral questioning over written testing is that the teacher knows immediately whether the learner understands the question and the teacher can let the learner know immediately whether the answer is right. In a group-teaching situation this kind of direct interchange is limited—although the reaction of one learner responding to another learner's answer can be very educational. In large groups the advantages

Box 3-4	*Cord Rating Scale*				

Score	Redness	Discharge	Odor	Dryness	Other/Comments
0	None	None	None	Hard	
1	Within $1/8$-inch of cord		Yes	Drying	
2	Within $1/4$-inch of cord	Reddish discharge		Soft, moist	
3	Within $1/2$-inch of cord	Yellowish discharge		Wet	

Note: It is normal to have a scant amount of bleeding from the cord site if the cord stump sticks to the diaper.

   MUST have a score of 7-10 for infection.

   Pustules present?

   _____ Yes

   _____ No

If yes, how long have they been present? _____

Where located? _____

Reprinted with permission from AWHONN © 1999. From Ford LA, Ritchie JA: Maternal perceptions of newborn umbilical cord treatments and healing, *J Obstet Gynecol Neonatal Nurs* 28:501-506, 1999.

of oral questioning are somewhat lost because every individual cannot respond to an oral question unless that response is in writing.

The verbal nature of both oral and written questioning may handicap individuals who have difficulty expressing themselves. Many individuals probably find it easier to express themselves orally than in writing. In addition, those who are verbally fluent may seem to know more. For these reasons, combinations of methods, such as observation of behavior and oral questioning, can often provide a truer picture than a single method can.

It is a common misconception that oral questioning does not require much preparation on the part of a teacher. Questions must be very carefully phrased so that (1) a learner can understand them and (2) they test the objective. Questions need to be carefully phrased to avoid leading a patient to the socially desirable answer or to "the answer" the provider wants, which may be an inappropriate reiteration of the information just presented by the provider. Such a circumstance may indicate that a patient has not comprehended the material well enough to express the idea in alternative ways.

Written Measurement

Written measurement is indirect and demands at least some reading skill and knowledge of test taking on the part of a learner.

Tests are prepared by individuals or groups of teachers in a particular institution and are used within that institution. They may be adapted to and published by other institutions, or they may be developed by test experts and sold. Tests sold commercially should provide a manual with information that explains the purposes of the test. Also, the manual should give evidence that the test accurately measures the goals it claims to measure and that it does so reliably. Evidence should include information that describes how well the test covers the subject matter. If, for example, the test is meant to evaluate knowledge of nutrition, it should include items on all the major concepts in nutrition today. This quality of a test is called content validity. Additional information should describe how closely the test score is related to actual patient behavior in the present (concurrent validity) or the future (predictive validity). For example, if a patient with diabetes scores high on the test, is he or she giving good self-care now? Will he or she be giving good self-care in the future? A similar kind of statement about future self-care would be needed for those doing less well on the test. If evidence from use of a test supports a high degree of validity, its value for decision making is greater than one for which little such information exists.

Only rarely are locally developed tests studied this carefully. Teachers who use their own tests and have continuing contact with the same patients gain a feeling for how closely the test relates to their patients' actual behavior. However, these teachers rarely perform studies that provide them with accurate test validity information. Measurement characteristics of more than 70 tools used in patient education may be found in Redman.[12] Several sample tools may be found on the following pages. The Chicago Lead Knowledge Test can be used to evaluate lead education programs (Box 3-5). (One group of parents in Chicago knew the answers to about half of these questions.)[11]

Box 3-5	*Chicago Lead Knowledge Test: Questions and Responses*[*]			
		Responses (percentage)		
Question	**Correct Answer**	**Correct**	**Incorrect**	**Don't Know**
General Information				
1. Lead paint chips can be poisonous when eaten.	True	95	1	4
2. High blood lead level can affect a child's ability to learn.	True	92	1	7
3. Most children have symptoms right away if they have an elevated blood lead level.	False	58	7	35
4. Apartment owners are required to tell renters about known lead-containing paint in the apartment when a lease is signed.	True	43	14	43
5. A child's highest blood lead level generally occurs around 5 years of age.	False	18	12	70
Exposure				
6. Lead paint is more likely to be found in newer homes than in older homes.	False	88	5	7
7. Living in a building during renovation/remodeling can increase a child's exposure to lead.	True	87	2	11
8. One way for children to get lead poisoning is by having lead dust on their hands and then putting their hands in their mouths.	True	86	2	12
9. A child can become lead poisoned during exposure to lead-containing dust.	True	85	1	14
10. Some pottery imported from Mexico or other countries is not safe to use for cooking or eating because it contains lead.	True	73	2	25
11. Parents who work with lead at their jobs can bring lead home on their clothes.	True	69	5	26
12. The lead a pregnant woman takes into her body can be transferred to the unborn baby.	True	67	2	31

Box 3-5	*Chicago Lead Knowledge Test: Questions and Responses*—cont'd				

	Responses (percentage)			
Question	**Correct Answer**	**Correct**	**Incorrect**	**Don't Know**
13. Lead in soil cannot harm children.	False	65	4	31
14. Most cases of childhood lead poisoning are caused by drinking water that contains lead.	False	40	20	40
15. Most children get lead poisoning by breathing in lead, rather than by eating or swallowing lead.	False	30	24	46
16. Some herbal or traditional home remedies contain lead.	True	16	7	77
Prevention				
17. Washing a child's hands often helps prevent lead poisoning.	True	47	27	26
18. Warm tap water usually contains less lead than cold tap water.	False	39	6	55
19. Lead in water can be removed by boiling.	False	32	20	48
20. Cleaning a home with soap and water decreases the lead in the home more than dusting or sweeping.	True	32	34	34
Nutrition				
21. The human body needs a small amount of lead for good nutrition.	False	27	17	56
22. Less lead is taken up by the body if a child eats a balanced diet, without too many fatty foods.	True	13	26	61
23. A diet with a good amount of iron-containing foods will help decrease a child's chance of becoming lead poisoned.	True	12	39	49
24. A diet with enough calcium helps prevent lead poisoning.	True	9	29	62

*In the survey, questions were ordered as follows: 6, 2, 1, 5, 3, 7, 17, 20, 23, 8, 19, 14, 18, 4, 11, 13, 10, 9, 12, 16, 15, 21, 24, 22.

From Mehta S, Binns HJ: What do parents know about lead poisoning? *Arch Pediatr Adolesc Med* 152:1213-1218, 1998.

The Diabetes Knowledge Questionnaire, shown in both English and Spanish, may be seen in Box 3-6. It was designed to assess overall diabetes knowledge according to content recommendations in the National Standards for Diabetes Patient Education Programs and was written in simple language to aid translation into the dialect of Spanish used by the population in Starr County, Texas. The instrument was first translated by regional native and bilingual speakers and then back-translated for accuracy and clarity. Content validity of the items was established by a panel of experienced nurses and researchers familiar with diabetes-related issues of Mexican-Americans. Further information about psychometric characteristics of this instrument may be found in Garcia and others.[3]

Sample items from a scale to measure the performance and frequency of self-care actions specific to patients with chronic obstructive

Box 3-6	*Diabetes Knowledge Questionnaire*			
Item #	Preguntas Questions	Si Yes	No No	No sé I don't know
1.	El comer mucha azúcar y otras comidas dulces es una cause de la diabetes.		√	
1.	Eating too much sugar and other sweet foods is a cause of diabetes.		√	
2.	La causa común de la diabetes es la falta de insulina efectiva en el cuerpo.	√		
2.	The usual cause of diabetes is lack of effective insulin in the body.	√		
3.	La diabetetes es causada porque los riñones no pueden mantener el azúcar fuera de la orina.		√	
3.	Diabetes is caused by failure of the kidneys to keep sugar out of the urine.		√	
4.	Los riñones producer la insulina.		√	
4.	Kidneys produce insulin.		√	
5.	En la diabetes que no se está tratando, la cantidad de azúcar en la sangre usualmente sube.	√		
5.	In untreated diabetes, the amount of sugar in the blood usually increases.	√		
6.	Si yo soy diabético, mis hijos tendran más riesgo de ser diábeticos.	√		
6.	If I am diabetic, my children have a higher chance of being diabetic.	√		
7.	Se puede curar la diabetes.		√	
7.	Diabetes can be cured.		√	
8.	Un nivel de azucar de 210 en prueba de sangre hecha en ayunas es muy alto.	√		
8.	A fasting blood sugar level of 210 is too high.	√		
9.	La mejor manera de checar mi diabetes es haciendo pruebas de orina.		√	
9.	The best way to check my diabetes is by testing my urine.		√	
10.	El ejercicio regular aumentará la necesidad de insulina u otro medicamento para la diabetes.		√	
10.	Regular exercise will increase the need for insulin or other diabetic medication.		√	
11.	Hay dos tipos principales de diabetes: tipo 1 (dependiente de insulina) y tipo 2 (no-dependiente de insulina).	√		
11.	There are two main types of diabetes: type 1 (insulin-dependent) and type 2 (non-insulin-dependent).	√		
12.	Una reacción de insulina es causada por mucha comida.		√	
12.	An insulin reaction is caused by too much food.		√	
13.	La medicina es más importante que la dieta y el ejercicio pare controlar mi diabetes.		√	
13.	Medication is more important than diet and exercise to control my diabetes.		√	

| Box 3-6 | *Diabetes Knowledge Questionnaire—cont'd* | | | |

Item #	Preguntas Questions	Si Yes	No No	No sé I don't know
14.	La diabetes frequentemente cause mala circulación.	√		
14.	Diabetes often causes poor circulation.	√		
15.	Cortaduras y rasguños cicatrizan mas despacio en diabéticos.	√		
15.	Cuts and abrasions on diabetics heal more slowly.	√		
16.	Los diabéticos deberían poner cuidado extra al cortarse las uñas de los dedos de los pies.	√		
16.	Diabetics should take extra care when cutting their toenails.	√		
17.	Una persona con diabetes debería limpiar una cortadura primero yodo y alcohol.		√	
17.	A person with diabetes should cleanse a cut with iodine and alcohol.		√	
18.	La manera en que preparo mi comida es igual de importante que las comidas que como.	√		
18.	The way I prepare my food is as important as the foods I eat.	√		
19.	La diabetes puede dañar mis riñones.	√		
19.	Diabetes can damage my kidneys.	√		
20.	La diabetes puede causer que no sienta en mis manos, dedos y pies.	√		
20.	Diabetes can cause loss of feeling in my hands, fingers, and feet.	√		
21.	El temblar y sudar son señales de azúcar alta en la sangre.		√	
21.	Shaking and sweating are signs of high blood sugar.		√	
22.	El orinar seguido y la sed son señales de azúcar baja en la sangre.		√	
22.	Frequent urination and thirst are signs of low blood sugar.		√	
23.	Los calcetines y las medias elásticas apretadas no son malos para los diabéticos.		√	
23.	Tight elastic hose or socks are not bad for diabetics.		√	
24.	Una dicta diabética consiste principalmente de comidas especiales.		√	
24.	A diabetic diet consists mostly of special foods.		√	

From Garcia AA, Villagomex ET, Brown SA, Kouzekanani K, Hanis CL. The Starr County diabetes education study, *Diabetes Care* 24:16-21, 2001. Copyright © 2001 American Diabetes Association. Reprinted with permission.

pulmonary disease (COPD) may be found in Box 3-7. Reported self-care actions are another example of outcomes that may be achieved by patient education. A final example of a written instrument is one that measures perceived confidence in diabetes self-care (frequently called self-efficacy) in persons with type 1 diabetes. Although self-efficacy is not the only explanatory factor in adequate self-care, it can add substantially to understanding of these behaviors (Box 3-8).

In some instances, no appropriate instrument will be available, and items to measure patient progress and outcomes must be constructed. Although multiple-choice, true-false, and matching items can be used, they may not provide accurate

Box 3-7	*Sample Questions from the COPD Self-Care Action Scale*					
		Frequency*				
Item		**Never**	**Rarely**	**Sometimes**	**Often**	**Very Often**
How often do you cut down on things you usually do because of shortness of breath?		————	————	————	————	————
How often do you get enough sleep and rest?		————	————	————	————	————
If you develop signs of an infection, how often do you report it to your doctor?		————	————	————	————	————
How often do you keep up with the air quality index or air pollution count report?		————	————	————	————	————
When you become suddenly short of breath, how often do you change your position?		————	————	————	————	————
When you are short of breath, how often do you sit on the edge of a chair, leaning forward?		————	————	————	————	————

*Responses are assigned numeric values: 0 = *never*, 1 = *rarely*, 2 = *sometimes*, 3 = *often*, 4 = *very often*.
From Riley P: Development of a COPD self-care action scale, *Rehabil Nurs Res* 5:3-8, 1996.

Box 3-8	*Confidence in Diabetes Self-Care Scale*

I believe I can …
  plan my meals and snacks according to dietary guidelines.
  check my blood glucose levels at least two times a day.
  perform the prescribed number of daily insulin injections.
  adjust my insulin for exercise, traveling, or celebrations.
  adjust my insulin when I am sick.
  detect high levels of blood glucose in time to correct.
  detect low levels of blood glucose in time to correct.
  treat a high blood glucose level correctly.
  treat a low blood glucose level correctly.
  keep daily records of my blood glucose levels.
  decide when it's necessary to contact my doctor or diabetes educator.
  ask my doctor questions about my treatment plan.
  keep my blood glucose in the normal range when under stress.
  check my feet for sores or blisters every day.
  ask my friends or relatives for help with my diabetes.
  inform colleagues/others of my diabetes, if needed.
  keep my medical appointments.
  exercise two to three times weekly.
  figure out what foods to eat when dining out.
  read and hear about diabetes complications without getting discouraged.
Scoring for each item from 1 ("No, I am sure I cannot") to 5 ("Yes, I am sure I can").

From Van Der Ven NCW and others: The confidence in diabetes self-care scale, *Diabetes Care* 26:713-718, 2003.

assessments for persons with marginal literacy. Short questions may be asked in oral or written form. An example is "What should be done if your child eats poison, and why should it be done?" Note that this question, whether oral or written, requires recall of information. However, the response will elicit a different behavior than does discriminating among answers that are already present in multiple-choice, true-false, and matching items.

The ability to recall is desirable for information used frequently. It is essential for emergency situations, such as child poisoning, diabetic coma, or seizures. The objective is to be able to recall the information and then act on it. A person must be able to produce the information from memory, not just recognize it among several alternatives. Periodic self-testing of memory for specific information will strengthen retention of infrequently used material. The strength of the recognition item is that it can enable learners to discriminate between ideas—ideas they might not otherwise consider—thus helping them test their depth of understanding.

Numerous possible errors in the construction of single test items and groups of items can prevent an accurate assessment of an individual's cognitive skills. For open-ended questions the provider can develop criteria for correct responses, ensuring consistency in scoring answers. Remember that guessing without really knowing the correct answer can inflate scores from true-false tests; some say this weakness should rule out their being used. Box 3-9 lists guidelines for writing multiple-choice test items. Note that multiple-choice items may have high complexity and readability levels and thus be very difficult for individuals with limited formal education to understand. Clues and implausible distractors help learners choose the correct answer by guessing, and thus they appear to know more than they do. By contrast, ambiguity makes it difficult for learners to demonstrate the knowledge they actually have. Testing for trivia may reliably provide information, but it is information about unimportant learning. Such errors should be avoided.

Box 3-10 provides an example of an asthma knowledge quiz, with correct responses in boldface. Critique this test for construction errors. Although most of the guidelines in Box 3-9 are met, all answers are choices b or c, which creates a clue. A few of the distractors are not very plausible. The "I don't know" response is not meant to be scored but to indicate areas where the parent needs instruction. Which of the items in Box 3-10 are so crucial that every parent must get them correct?

Test theorists suggest generating a number of items representing a domain (an objective) and randomly drawing a sample of items from each domain.

EVALUATIVE JUDGMENTS

Measurement is carried out so that the teaching-learning process can be evaluated more accurately than it could be by general impressions. Evaluation must go beyond measurement. It requires a value judgment about learning and teaching. Evaluation must summarize the evidence and determine how well the objectives are being met.

Measurement and evaluation occur continuously during teaching, serving to redirect the activities of teachers and learners. Information about learners' progress is gathered by having learners respond to questions or perform periodically, or both. The expressions of boredom, interest, confusion, or enlightenment on learners' faces give clues about their understanding of the material being taught.

Some individuals are able to tell a teacher that they do not understand. Others cannot identify or express their uncertainty. To identify material that is not clear to learners, the provider can retrace the explanation or the skill demonstration, ask questions at intervals, or observe and critique the performance of a skill by a learner. This technique will point out terms used by the teacher that learners may not understand, or it may reveal that learners are overloaded with complex instructions. Trying to reteach without determining the nature of the learning problem may cause a caregiver to make the same error

Box 3-9	*A Revised Taxonomy of Multiple Choice Item-Writing Guidelines*

Content Concerns

1. Every item should reflect specific content and a single specific mental behavior, as called for in test specifications (two-way grid, test blueprint).
2. Base each item on important content to learn; avoid trivial content.
3. Use novel material to test higher level learning. Paraphrase textbook language or language used during instruction when used in a test item, to avoid testing for simple recall.
4. Keep the content of each item independent from content of other items on the test.
5. Avoid overspecific and over general content when writing MC items.
6. Avoid opinion-based items.
7. Avoid trick items.
8. Keep vocabulary simple for the group of students being tested.

Formatting Concerns

9. Use the question, completion, and best answer versions of the conventional MC, the alternate choice, true-false, multiple true-false, matching, and the context-dependent item and item set formats, but AVOID the complex MC (type K) format.
10. Format the item vertically instead of horizontally.

Style Concerns

11. Edit and proof items.
12. Use correct grammar, punctuation, capitalization, and spelling.
13. Minimize the amount of reading in each item.

Writing the Stem

14. Ensure that the directions in the stem are very clear.
15. Include the central idea in the stem instead of the choices.

16. Avoid window dressing (excess verbiage).
17. Word the step positively, avoid negatives such as NOT or EXCEPT. If negative words are used, use the word cautiously and always ensure that the word appears captitalized and boldfaced.

Writing the Choices

18. Develop as many effective choices as you can, but research suggests three is adequate.
19. Make sure that only one of these choices is the right answer.
20. Vary the location of the right answer according the number of choices.
21. Place choices in logical or numerical order.
22. Keep choices independent; choices should not be overlapping.
23. Keep choices homogenous in content and grammatical structure.
24. Keep the length of choices about equal.
25. *None-of-the-above* should be used carefully.
26. Avoid *All-of-the-above*.
27. Phrase choices positively; avoid negatives such as NOT.
28. Avoid giving clues to the right answer, such as
    a. Specific determiners including always, never, completely, and absolutely.
    b. Clang associations, choices identical to or resembling words in the stem.
    c. Grammatical inconsistencies that cue the test-taker to the correct choice.
    d. Conspicuous correct choice.
    e. Pairs or triplets of options that clue the test-taker to the correct choice.
    f. Blatantly absurd, ridiculous options.
29. Make all distractors plausible.
30. Use typical errors of students to write your distractors.
31. Use humor if it is compatible with the teacher and the learning environment.

MC, Multiple choice.
(From Haladyna TM, Downing SM, Rodriguez MC: A review of multiple-choice item-writing guidelines for classroom assessment. *Appl Meas Educ* 15:309-334, 2002.)

Box 3-10	*Asthma Knowledge Quiz Items*

1. If your child starts to wheeze badly and you give him/her a rescue medicine, how long should it take before he/she breathes better?
   a. 45 minutes
   b. 10 minutes
   c. 2 hours
   d. I don't know

2. What is the most important thing that your child should know?
   a. How to take medicines on his/her own
   b. To tell you when he/she has trouble breathing
   c. To stay away from strong odors
   d. I don't know

3. Antibiotics are drugs that work against
   a. Viruses only
   b. Bacteria only
   c. Viruses and bacteria
   d. I don't know

4. Usually someone gets asthma because
   a. Of stress
   b. Of pollution
   c. Of family characteristic
   d. I don't know

5. How should your child blow into a peak flow meter?
   a. Slowly, with lots of blows
   b. Slowly, with one long blow
   c. Quickly, with one hard blow
   d. I don't know

6. If your child has had an asthma attack, when is the best time to see a doctor again?
   a. The next time he/she has an attack
   b. When he/she is better
   c. At an annual checkup
   d. I don't know

7. Your child has trouble talking and you notice that his/her fingertips are blue; you should
   a. Give him/her his/her inhaler
   b. Take him/her to an emergency department
   c. Give him/her the inhaler and take him/her to an emergency department
   d. I don't know

8. What happens to the airways during an asthma attack?
   a. They fill with mucus
   b. They squeeze shut
   c. They squeeze shut and fill with mucus
   d. I don't know

9. When your child has his/her asthma under control:
   a. He /she will still have a lot of trouble breathing on occasion
   b. He/she will have some trouble breathing, but it is not very important
   c. He/she should not have any trouble breathing even if he/she runs a lot
   d. I don't know

10. If your child needs to use his/her inhaler seven times a day, you should
    a. Take him/her to an emergency department
    b. Call the doctor to adjust the medicines
    c. Let him/her use it up to 10 times a day
    d. I don't know

11. Your child can intentionally start an asthma attack
    a. True
    b. False
    c. I don't know

12. Which of the following is a trigger of asthma?
    a. Spicy foods
    b. Cat fur
    c. Loud sounds
    d. I don't know

From Jones JA and others: Increasing asthma knowledge and changing home environments for Latino families with asthmatic children, *Patient Educ Counseling* 42:67-79, 2001.

again. It is unwise to teach for a long time (or even one lesson period) without requiring learners to respond so that teaching and learning errors can be corrected.

Adequacy of learning must eventually be evaluated in terms of meeting the final objectives and commonly accepted outcomes. Of course, if satisfactory evaluation takes place as the teaching is going on, the degree of attainment of final objectives or the time needed to meet the final objectives can be quite accurately predicted (Box 3-11).

Box 3-11 | *Possible Errors in Teaching-Learning Process if Goals Are Not Being Met*

Readiness/Motivation Goals

1. Did the learner ever accept the goals, or were you teaching only what you believed to be important?
2. What evidence do you have that the goals were appropriate?
3. Were the goals clearly written and understood by teacher and learner?
4. Were the goals broken into sufficient intermediate steps to provide guidance?

Teaching-Learning

1. Had teaching materials previously been tried with persons of ability similar to that of your patient and found successful?
2. If previous experience with the materials was not available, in what ways did their characteristics match the patient's readiness?
3. Were evaluative data gathered often during teaching, to give evidence of areas of success and lack of success?
4. Was teaching continued for sufficient time for learning to be thorough?
5. Were the data gathered for evaluation sufficiently valid and reliable to form an adequate basis for the evaluative decision?
6. Were baseline data obtained for measuring change? People rarely start with no knowledge or skill.

Critical paths provide a structure of expected outcomes within particular time frames that guide all care, including patient education.

Crucial decisions regarding patients, such as whether living alone is likely to be safe, rest on the outcome of learning. The minimum performance necessary for an individual to function must be identified. Certain basic information and skills and a level of confidence must be learned because they are essential to the performance of a particular task. Other information and skills may also be crucial, depending on how independently the individual will be functioning. If crucial items are answered incorrectly, reteaching is necessary until the knowledge or skills are assured. Sometimes the learner becomes hostile, which may a way of expressing a desire to get out of the situation. Evidence of positive change in learners is rewarding for teachers as well as learners.

The relationship between a learner's competence and a teacher's competence is entangled in evaluation. To some extent this relationship depends on which person is regarded as more responsible for learning. Sometimes it is obvious that a teacher cannot communicate or does not understand the subject matter. In this case the teacher needs to be helped to develop teaching skill. Teaching has the potential for being both harmful and ineffective, and professional incompetence exists in this area of nursing or medicine as in any other area. Possible harmful effects of ineffective teaching include leaving a patient with incapacitating confusion, a loss of self-confidence, or an inability to accomplish necessary reintegration into a family or other social group.

Evaluation of teaching and learning also includes a perspective of the known limitations of teaching today—particularly in the area of motivating individuals. Knowledge of the determinants of behavior at the present time is both limited and fragmented, and practical means of assessing the relative influence of each factor are virtually nonexistent. Therefore, in a particular situation it is difficult to estimate how each factor that is already present is influencing particular behavior and how new factors might affect behavior. In many of the complex situations that require learning, reality factors, such as poverty, health, and family crisis, limit the effect that teaching can have. In such situations small, but important, effects are characteristic even of the "good" programs.

One solution has been to use several complementary kinds of interventions (teaching may be one) to maximize the effect. Sometimes nothing seems to have an effect, and an individual or family does not recover from illness or achieve high-level wellness. Explanation may be sought through inquiry into a patient's perceptions, motives, values, confidence, intelligence, grasp of relevant knowledge, and skills. It has also been suggested that a patient's situation might reflect a condition such as powerlessness, and his or her ability to learn may be only one of the behaviors affected.

SUMMARY

Although evaluation is the final step in the process of teaching-learning, it is forward-looking because its message redirects activity (Box 3-11). Information necessary for an evaluation of how well objectives have been met is gathered by various measurement techniques. A concerted effort is made to gather reliable information by perfecting measurement approaches and by using them in conjunction with one another. This method provides a sounder basis for decisions about the competence of the learner to function in the manner specified in the objectives.

Study Questions

1. You observe a nurse who has been teaching a patient how to give himself an injection. The nurse asks the patient the following questions as he goes through the procedure: Is it all right to give the injection with the same syringe and needle you used yesterday? Review why you are wiping the skin a particular way. What would you do if the tip of the needle touched the table as you were picking up the syringe? What would you do if you touched the skin now (after it has been cleansed with the alcohol sponge and before the injection is given)? State the subobjective that the nurse is evaluating.

2. How is the notion of transfer of learning used in evaluation?

3. You are trying to teach a mentally challenged youngster self-dressing skills, and he is inattentive and rebellious. It is obvious that he is showing lack of motivation to learn. List three possible factors that might be producing this behavior, and indicate the action a caregiver might take in response to each.

4. You are the teacher in a class for patients with diabetes who make the following comments. What evidence does each question or comment give about the individual's understanding?
   a. "Would blood sugar be the same for man, woman, or child?"
   b. "I don't feel I'm really a diabetic because I don't have to take insulin." (The patient is a 19-year-old woman in whom pregnancy-precipitated signs and symptoms of diabetes are being controlled by diet.)
   c. Father whose 8-year-old son has newly diagnosed diabetes, talking to a college student who has been insulin-dependent for 2 years: "Are you able to hunt?"

Box 3-12	*Format for Tunneled Central Line Care Stations*		
Station	**Content Area**	**Medium/Supplies**	**Examination**
A	Dressing change	Ned-Chest™ model Dressing change supplies	Skill demonstration
B	Moisture under dressing	Still-life colored photos	Identify problem and proposed action
C	Infected line	Still-life colored photos	Identify problem and proposed action

Box 3-12	*Format for Tunneled Central Line Care Stations—cont'd*

Station	Content Area	Medium/Supplies	Examination
D	Flushing line	Ned-Chest™ model Line-flushing supplies	Skill demonstration
E	Contamination during flushing	Video clip of contamination during flushing	Identify problem and proposed action
F	Cap change	Ned-Chest™ model Cap change supplies	Skill demonstration
G	Contamination during cap change	Video clip of contamination during cap change	Identify problem and proposed action

You have had no problems with the central line catheter. It is time for the routine dressing change.
1. How often do you change the dressing?
2. What would you do before you begin changing the dressing?
Here are the necessary supplies for a dressing change. At this time, show how you change the catheter dressing using the model chest with the central line.
Medium: Ned-Chest™ model with central line and dressing
Supplies: Towel or blue pad   Iodine swabs (1 Pkg)
              Gloves   Alcohol wipes (3)
              Alcohol swabs (1 Pkg)   IV-3000 dressing

Rating Form

	Evaluation Criteria	Yes	No
	Identify time interval for dressing change *Answer: every 5 days*		
	What would you do first? Or what would you do before you begin changing the dressing? *Answer: Wash hands*		
	Demonstration of Dressing Change		
	1. Remove old dressing		
	2. Wash hands again		
	3. Put on gloves		
Station A— tunneled central line dressing change.	4. Cleanse site:		
	Clean to dirty		
	Alcohol swab first		
	Then iodine swab		
	5. Cleanse line:		
	Clean to dirty		
	Alcohol wipes		
	6. Apply IV-3000:		
	Without stretching		
	Remove finger tabs		
	Reinforce with finger tabs		
	7. Discard used dressing/supplies		

From Heermann JA, Eilers JG, Carney PA: Use of modified OSCEs to verify technical skill performance and competency of lay caregivers, *J Cancer Educ* 16:93-98, 2001.

5. Demands on lay caregivers of blood and marrow stem cell transplant recipients are complex. To ensure their competence, Heerman, Eilers, and Carney[6] set up an objective, structured clinical examination with seven practice stations for the care of tunneled central lines. The lay caregivers must satisfactorily perform each of these tasks to be considered competent. The stations and evaluation criteria for station A may be seen in Box 3-12. Objective, structured clinical examinations are not common in patient education. Is this an appropriate evaluative approach?

REFERENCES

1. Clancy CM, Eisenberg JM: Outcomes research: measuring the end results of health care, *Science* 282: 245-246, 1998.

2. Ford LA, Ritchie JA: Maternal perceptions of newborn umbilical cord treatments and healing, *J Obstet Gynecol Neonatal Nurs* 28:501-506, 1999.

3. Garcia HA, Villagomez ET, Brown SA, Kouzekanani K, Hanis CL: The Starr County diabetes education study, *Diabetes Care* 24:16-21, 2001.

4. Glasgow RE: Outcomes of and for diabetes education research, *Diabetes Educator* 25(suppl):74-88, 1999.

5. Haladyna TM, Downing SM, Rodriguez MC: A review of multiple-choice item-writing guidelines for classroom assessment. *Appl Meas Educ* 15:309-334, 2002.

6. Heerman JA, Eilers JG, Carney PA: Use of modified OSCEs to verify technical skill performance and competency of law caregivers. *J Cancer Educ* 16:93-98, 2001.

7. Holmes-Rovner M and others: Patient satisfaction with health care decisions, *Med Decis Making* 16:58-64, 1996.

8. Johnson M, Maas M, editors: *Classification of nursing outcomes*, St. Louis, 1997, Mosby.

9. Jones JA and others: Increasing asthma knowledge and changing home environments for Latino families with asthmatic children. *Pat Educ Counsel* 42:67-79, 2001.

10. Lorig K and others: *Outcome measures for health education and other health care interventions*, Thousand Oaks, CA, 1996, Sage.

11. Mehta S, Binns HJ: What do parents know about lead poisoning? *Arch Pediatr Adolesc Med* 152:1213-1218, 1998.

12. Redman BK: *Measurement tools in patient education*, ed 2. New York, 2003, Springer.

13. Riley P: Development of a COPD self-care action scale, *Rehabil Nurs Res* 5:3-8, 1996.

14. Van der Ven NCW and others: The confidence in diabetes self-care scale. *Diab Care* 26:713-718, 2003.

15. Wood RY: Reliability and validity of a breast self examination proficiency rating instrument, *Eval Health Prof* 17:418-435, 1994.

Cancer Patient Education

GENERAL APPROACH

Education helps individuals detect their own cancer and aids in treatment and rehabilitation. Perhaps the greatest effort in cancer education has been placed on teaching self-assessment techniques such as breast self-examination and on persuading individuals to seek other screening techniques such as Papanicolaou (Pap) smears or colon cancer screening. Because minority women are more likely to seek medical care when breast and cervical cancers are in an advanced stage,[1] special attention is being paid to cultural models for assessing how individuals from these populations understand cancer and how interventions can best be delivered to them. Because cancer is a chronic disease, the needs of families and home caregivers and the use of cancer support groups have also received attention, as has the education necessary to adequately manage pain associated with the disease. Americans' knowledge about major risk factors and survival after early detection for common cancers (breast, cervical, and colon) is poor for all ages and races. Those at greatest risk—the oldest—have the least knowledge.[3] Increasing accuracy of risk perception is important.

EDUCATIONAL APPROACHES

Patient confusion over basic cancer terminology suggests that routine reporting and debriefing mechanisms in patient care should be reformed. For example, reports sent to women indicating that their cervical smear was negative do not communicate clearly that the test was "normal." Such reports should be accompanied by a sentence stating that this report means you have low risk for development of cervical cancer in the next 5 years.[23] Likewise, the term "dyskariosis" is used in cytology to describe nuclear abnormalities in cervical cells and is the basis for referral for colposcopy. Because of their lack of knowledge of the meaning of this term, women often assume they have cancer. They also needed information about what happens during colposcopy and possible side effects.[25] Box 4-1 provides sensory information for colposcopy. Sensory as well as procedural information has in general been found to improve preparation for a procedure and to speed recovery.

Concerns that teaching self-screening and encouraging its practice will raise anxiety were not supported in a study of testicular self-examination in young men.[33] More complex relationships among anxiety and skill, confidence, and adherence to breast self-examination (BSE) are documented in recent literature. As many as half of women with a family history of breast cancer have persistent distress related to their increased risk, with these feelings beginning as early as adolescence. Some overestimate their risk by as much as four times their actual risk. Lower rates of self-screening were found in women who were more distressed. Coming to terms with this risk requires information and

---

Box 4-1	*Sensory Information Message for Colposcopy*

Once you have changed into a hospital gown for the procedure, you will be taken to the colposcopy room. In the room, you will notice an examining table with stirrups, a cart holding instruments, and the colposcope (a piece of equipment that looks like a microscope). You will be asked to get up on the examining table and to slide down on the table so that your feet are in the stirrups. A clinician will explain the procedure to you either before it is done or as it is being done.

The clinician may perform a pelvic examination. Then, he/she inserts a speculum, which will feel cool and uncomfortable. Once the speculum is in place, the clinician will clean and examine your cervix. He/she also will apply vinegar to your cervix. The vinegar helps the clinician to see any abnormal area(s) better. The vinegar will feel cool.

The clinician may take a sample of secretions from your cervical canal. This means that he/she will quickly move a probe in and out of the cervix. If this is part of your examination, you will feel a cramping sensation that will last as long as it takes to obtain the sample.

The clinician will take a biopsy specimen of any abnormal area(s) on the cervix. You will likely hear a snipping sound as the clamps come together and feel a pinch as the biopsy is being taken. The pinching sensation lasts only seconds.

The clinician will remove the speculum, which will give you a sense of relief. It may seem as though the speculum is being removed more slowly than it is when you have a Pap test. The reason for the difference is that the clinician can use the colposcope to take a good look at the top part of your vagina.

The clinician may also examine your external genitals. If this is part of your examination, he/she will spray vinegar on this area so that any abnormal area(s) are seen more easily. The vinegar will feel cool.

The procedure is now completed. You are asked to sit up on the side of the examining table. You will be given information about how and when you will receive the biopsy results.

Reprinted with permission from AWHONN © 1999. From Nugent LS, Clark CR; Colposcopy: sensory information for client education, *Obstet Gynecol* 25:225-231, 1996.

support.[7,19] A randomized controlled trial (RCT) testing messages tailored specifically to the subject's stage of adoption of mammography by use of the transtheoretical model (see Chapter 1) along with basic education about breast cancer risk significantly reduced womens' risk overestimate.[9] Not doing BSE or doing it irregularly can allow women to maintain control over their feelings of threat.

Demonstration as a method of teaching BSE is insufficient. Actual practice in developing tactile skill in detecting abnormalities must lead to competence and confidence. For women who did not feel competent of their ability to detect lumps, self-examination served to increase their feelings of being "out of control" with a resultant increase in anxiety. Women who rate their ability to self-examine highly have been found to be more likely to carry out regular BSE and to act on abnormalities they may find.[6]

When there are many equivalent options for a single problem, formal decision aids have been found to be useful for establishing patient preferences. Figure 4-1 shows an example of a decision board to assist women with lymph node–positive breast cancer to choose between two adjuvant

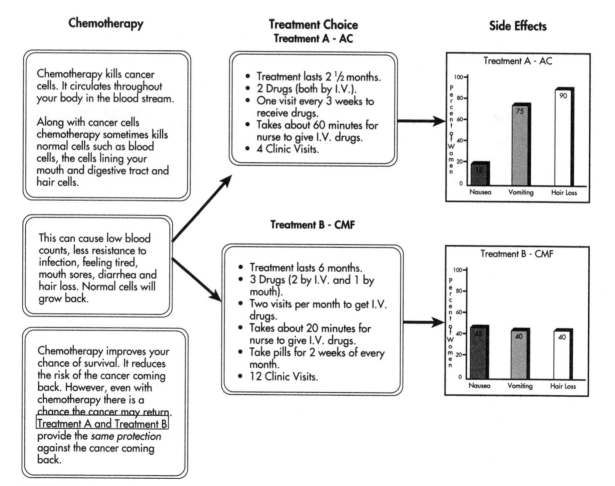

FIGURE 4-1 Schematic depiction of the decision board. (From Irwin E and others: Offering a choice between two adjuvant chemotherapy regimens: a pilot study to develop a decision aid for women with breast cancer, *Patient Educ Couns* 37:283-291, 1999.)

chemotherapy treatments. The clinician reads the written material aloud and explains the graphic material contained on seven cards and placed on the board in sequence.[18] A similar decision aid (this time in the form of an audiotape and workbook) has been developed for women facing surgical treatment of early-stage breast cancer by breast-conserving therapy or mastectomy. Because these treatments have been found to yield equal outcomes, patients may need assistance in considering their choices. Decision aids differ from traditional educational materials in their emphasis on alternatives, detailed descriptions of risks and benefits, and frequently values clarification exercises.[29]

A similar approach can be used for men considering screening for prostate cancer. A recent study found well-educated men to be not well informed about the natural history of prostate cancer, the benefits of treatment, or the predictive value of prostate-specific antigen (PSA) tests—all important factors to understand before they can participate meaningfully in a decision about screening. Participation is particularly important because personal preferences of well-informed men have been found to be evenly divided between accepting or forgoing screening.[14]

Family support in dealing with cancer is also necessary. Several longitudinal studies of patients and spouses indicate that the stressful effects of cancer extend as long as 1 to 2 years after the initial diagnosis. For the most part, spouses report receiving little information about their partner's illness, and their attempts to request information or to contact the physician by telephone were often unsuccessful. It is believed that families need a framework of expectations about the emotional aspects of recovery that can serve as a measure against which they can monitor progress and receive encouragement to view their concerns as a normal part of the recovery process.[26] A home-based educational program for family caregivers of cancer patients who receive hospice and home care provided videotapes of physical care procedures such as safe transfer for bed to chair along with a videotape on understanding common emotions and communicating with children about cancer.[27] The video of care

procedures allows repeated reviewing; one would hope that it is accompanied by supervised skill building. Patients with advanced cancer have complicated medical problems that require multiple treatments or diagnostic interventions; they have a high frequency of debilitating symptoms such as pain, nausea, cachexia, depression, and anxiety; and they frequently misinterpret information they received during their oncology visits. Audiotapes added to written materials after a provider visit have been shown to improve patients' specific knowledge about what was discussed and recommended.[5]

Educational interventions for pain management are important because pain affects 50% to 80% of patients with cancer and is poorly controlled in an estimated 80%. PRO-SELF interventions have been well studied. An RCT testing the module on pain control showed a clinically significant decrease in pain from baseline for the majority of patients in comparison with those in a comparison group. A PRO-SELF nurse coached patients on how to improve pain relief by altering times and frequency of analgesic intake while staying within the prescription, how to assess pain and their responses to analgesia, strategies to prevent or treat analgesic side effects, and how to speak with their providers if the analgesic prescription was not adequate. Patients were taught to use a pill box and were coached during two follow-up phone visits.[24] A smaller study with less intensive intervention (10 to 15 minutes per day for 5 days) showed significantly less pain intensity and negative beliefs about opioids and less pain catastrophizing.[20] Other studies have used personalized pain management plans and coaching to assist patients to learn more adaptive ways to communicate pain.[34]

Patients have educational needs at all stages of cancer diagnosis and treatment. Women whose breast biopsy specimens show benign conditions still require education to answer questions such as, What is fibrocystic disease? Will benign breast disease turn into cancer?[10] Likewise, long-term survivors of breast cancer frequently are confused about what is adequate follow-up once cancer treatment ends. They want information about how to monitor their own bodies and how to manage symptoms such as lymphedema.[15] Lethborg and Kissane[22] describe a post–adjuvant treatment support program for the period after treatment ends. Psychoeducation at this stage can include stress management, enhancement of coping skills, increase in confidence for dealing with anxiety, and general health education.

In addition to instrumental learning such as information about pain management, persons with cancer and their families struggle to establish meaning about what is happening to them. In life-threatening illness, meaning affects coping behavior, has an impact on psychosocial well-being, and is important in the struggle to obtain a sense of mastery. Meaning refers to an individual's understanding of the implications an illness has for his or her identity and for the future—perceptions of the ability to accomplish future goals, to maintain the viability of interpersonal relationships, and to sustain a sense of personal vitality, competence, and power. The constructed meaning scale, shown in Box 4-2, is a measure of

Box 4-2	*Constructed Meaning Scale*

1. I feel cancer is something I will never recover from.
2. I feel cancer is serious, but I will be able to return to life as it was before my illness.
3. I feel cancer has changed my life permanently so it will never be as good again.
4. I feel I have made a complete recovery from my illness.
5. I feel that I am the same person as I was before my illness.
6. I feel that my relationships with other people have not been negatively affected by my illness.
7. I feel that my experience with cancer has made me a better person.
8. I feel that having cancer has interfered with my achievement of the most important goals I have set for myself.

From Fife BL: The measurement of meaning in illness, *Soc Sci Med* 40:1021-1028, 1995.

such meaning. Each statement allows a response on a scale of 1 to 4: strongly disagree, disagree, agree, or strongly agree. The lowest test score, 9, indicates a very negative sense of the meaning the illness holds for one's self and for one's future. The authors discuss the validity and reliability in the text of their article.[12]

A number of measurement tools that may be used in clinical practice or research are presented and reviewed in Redman.[28] Instruments are available to assess informational needs of patients with breast cancer and colorectal cancer.

COMMUNITY-BASED EDUCATION AND EDUCATION OF SPECIAL POPULATIONS

Teaching tools for the education of patients with cancer are widely available from national voluntary and government agencies. As with other areas of practice, there are very few materials written at lower reading levels. Teaching tools are published regularly in professional journals, such as *Oncology Nursing Forum*, *Journal of the American Medical Association*, and *Nurse Practitioner*, which serve to educate the professional nursing community so that practitioners can fulfill their patient education roles.

Genetic testing to identify high risk for certain cancers such as those of the breast or ovary brings its own set of educational challenges. In general, women are better educated about breast cancer than they are about genetic testing. Many women want to have genetic testing without understanding the full ramifications of the decision process. Women at high risk who decline may be at increased risk for depression even more than those found to be gene-mutation carriers. Women with less than high school education had less knowledge of genetic testing than did others, yet were more willing to undergo it.[20]

The educational needs of a number of special populations with cancer require attention. For example, more than 50% of all cancers occur in the 11% of the population older than 65 years of age; yet very little attention has been paid to the educational needs of this population. Mortality caused by cancer is higher in minority groups, partially because some ethnic groups are less aware of the signs and symptoms of cancer and may have beliefs that are divergent from the mainstream of the health care system. Each major ethnic population serves as an identifying category for several diverse populations within it. It is important to look at cancer knowledge, beliefs, and attitudes by socioeconomic status as well as by cultural group. In addition, research has shown that different ethnic groups have different styles of learning. Most efforts to meet the educational and informational needs of different ethnic groups have revolved around translated materials, focus groups conducted to ensure cultural relevance, and community leadership involvement.

A study of low-income African-American women older than 40 years of age in Atlanta, Georgia, found that their cancer models differed significantly from those held by clinicians.[16] The women attending these clinics endured cancer-screening tests that to them seemed to serve only as heralds of a disease that would ultimately kill them and that was outside the realm of physicians' abilities. Many women preferred to remain ignorant of the existence of cancer. Many believed that cancer originates as a bruise or sore that will not heal. Almost 60% believed that surgery just makes the cancer worse by exposing the tumor to air and thereby spreading the disease. Faith in God seemed to be one of the few completely benign and truly powerful treatment alternatives available to an individual with cancer. Given the explanatory models of this group of women, the question to ask is why any women in this group would undergo screening.

An excellent example of a culturally relevant educational approach gives information about cervical health in a game format called Loteria, which is familiar to many adult Hispanic women of Mexican descent.[30] As in the traditional Loteria game, pictures are matched with written text that instructs them about the risk factors for cervical cancer, screening guidelines for cervical cancer, and the increased rate for invasive cervical cancer found in adult Hispanic women. Because many members of the target population did not have transportation outside their community, the educational programs were presented in churches, clubs, and clinics, with gifts of cosmetics supplied to participants. The importance of staying well by undergoing regular Pap testing was highlighted as allowing the women to continue to perform their roles as mother and wife, important in the Hispanic culture.

A program to increase prostate cancer screening in African-American men found that a peer educator method (testimony by African-American men in support of prostate cancer screening) and phone calls aimed at removing screening barriers or reminders for screening were more effective than was "standard education." This population can often be more easily recruited into work sites, churches, housing projects, or barbershops than into health care settings. The men in this study needed to understand the absence of symptoms in early stages of prostate cancer and the various treatment options available.[32]

"Witnessing," in which role models who have survived cancer tell of their experiences in groups at churches and community organizations, is well matched to certain cultures. One group of African American women did not know that mammography was associated with cancer, confused it with a Pap smear, and believed that the test was not necessary if their breasts were smaller or felt fine.[11] Cervical cancer screen-ing education culturally acceptable for American Indian women used talking circles, in which each member provides a 5- to 10-minute story sharing information and support.[17] This culture has a strong oral tradition and a strong sense of privacy. Table 4-1 provides a list of breast cancer educational materials useful for this population.[4]

CASE II

Because chemotherapy treatment for women with breast cancer is frequently provided on an ambulatory outpatient basis, side effects are likely to be encountered at home. Some patients are vulnerable to the development of anticipatory nausea and vomiting (ANV), likely based on classical conditioning, in which nausea and vomiting induced by the chemotherapy experience become linked with other stimuli such as smells, memories, and visual cues (the conditioned stimulus). The giving of accurate, realistic, and understandable information is paramount

TABLE 4-1 American Indian and Low Literacy Breast Cancer Education Materials		
Educational Materials	**Description**	**Availability**
American Indian		
"Circle of Life: A Breast Cancer Awareness Project for American Indian Women" educational kit	This train-the-trainer kit includes American Indian designs and artwork on flip charts, brochures, and a teacher's and trainer's manual.	American Cancer Society, Oklahoma Division
"How to Examine Your Breasts" poster	The poster depicts an American Indian shield with a step-by-step illustration of BSE.	National American Women's Health Education Resource Center, Lake Andes, SD
"Malam Nau Yahiwapo: Women's Gathering Place" folder and fact sheets	The decorative folder contains fact sheets about breast health, clinical breast examination, BSE, and mammography (ninth grade reading level).	Arizona Disease Prevention Center, Tucson, Ariz
"We are the Circle of Life: Pass on the Gift of Health" poster	The poster depicts an artistic drawing of four American Indian women, with the caption "Get yearly mammograms and Pap screenings."	American Indian Health Care Association, St Paul, Minn.
"Continue the Circle: Enjoy the Gift of Health" mammogram poster	The poster depicts three American Indian women from three generations, with the caption "Please get a mammogram."	American Cancer Society, Minneapolis, Minn
"What Women Should Know About Cancer" brochure	The brochure discusses the early signs of breast and other cancers and contains seven easy-to-read comics.	American Cancer Society, Eureka, Calif
"Breast Cancer: Know the Facts—A Situation No Woman Wants to Face" brochure	The brochure contains information about breast cancer and recommended screening guidelines, with American Indian art on the cover (ninth grade reading level).	American Indian Women's Health Education Resource Center, Lake Andes, SD
Low Literacy		
"A Mammogram Could Save Your Life" brochure	The brochure stresses the importance of mammography and answers questions about the procedure.	National Cancer Institute, Bethesda, Md
"Take Care of Your Breasts" brochure	The brochure defines mammography and provides guidelines for mammography screening.	National Cancer Institute, Bethesda, Md
"Breast Cancer Questions and Answers" pamphlet	The pamphlet answers nine basic questions about breast cancer.	American Cancer Society, Atlanta, Ga
"Woman to Woman: Straight Talk About Mammography" video	The video depicts older women of all races voicing their concerns about mammography.	American Cancer Society, Atlanta, Ga

From Bront JM, Fallsdown D, Iverson ML: The evolution of a breast health program for plains Indian women, *Oncol Nurs Forum* 26:731-739, 1999.

in empowering patients and enhancing their individual coping. One means to do this is a patient information leaflet (PIL).

To describe their needs, seven women in a breast cancer support group were convened to discuss possible content for a PIL for ANV. The PIL had three main aims:

1. to inform women about ANV and help them to identify the problem
2. to encourage women to raise the issue with their health care teams and get further help in managing the problem, and
3. to give women some ideas and methods to control their symptoms and improve their sense of well-being and empowerment during the process.

The designed PIL was evaluated by other women with breast cancer on criteria of comprehensibility, length, relevance, and presentation; they were also asked to add any important omitted information. The PIL's reading ease was rated as standard. The majority of women noted reassurance from identification of the problem and normalizing feelings. There is now a need to evaluate how the PIL is being used by women who experience ANV, for example, in seeking help in enhancing self-management.[2]

How would you evaluate this work?

SUMMARY

Goals in education for patients with cancer include helping the patient adjust to the course of the disease, carry out self-care and prescribed regimens, recognize and control side effects, achieve a sense of participation in and control over care, and normalize lifestyle and interactions—all discussed in the preceding examples of educational interventions in institutional and community settings and with varied populations. It is important to note that far more research and educational program development seem to be focused on breast and, to a lesser extent, cervical cancer than on other equally important neoplastic diseases, although the general principles of screening, self-care, coping, and family support are applicable to all.

Study Questions

1. Box 4-3 provides an example of a test for breast cancer risk assessment. Provide a critique of the test.

Box 4-3	*True-or-False Questions*

1. A woman's risk of breast cancer remains the same throughout her lifetime. (False)
2. For most women, the ordinary lumpiness they feel in their breasts does not increase their risk of breast cancer. (True)
3. Most women who develop breast cancer do not have any known risk factors. (True)
4. Most breast cancers are inherited. (False)
5. All known risk factors for breast cancer are included in the Gail Model. (False)
6. The medication tamoxifen can decrease the risk of breast cancer for women who are at increased risk for development of the disease. (True)
7. Tamoxifen should be prescribed for all women at increased risk for breast cancer. (False)
8. Raloxifene is approved for the treatment of osteoporosis and is being studied for use in breast cancer prevention. (True)
9. Most advances in breast cancer are the result of knowledge gained through clinical trials. (True)
10. A woman getting regular mammograms need not have clinical breast examinations. (False)

(From Snyder LA others, Development of the breast cancer education and risk assessment program, *Oncol Nurs Forum* 30:803-808, 2003.)

2. The following questions were found on an instrument to measure patient knowledge about cancer: "Do you know how to examine your breasts?" "Do you know where your prostate gland is located in your body?"[13] Will these items yield valid answers?
3. An educational session on BRCA1/2 testing addresses the following topics: (1) inheritance of susceptibility to breast-ovarian cancer, (2) cancer risks associated with BRCA1 or BRCA2 mutations, (3) genetic linkage studies, gene identification, and tests for mutation status, (4) benefits of genetic testing including the potential for early detection and reduction of uncertainty, (5) limitations of genetic testing

How To Do Breast Self-Examination

Do breast self-examination (BSE) every month. Become familiar with how your breasts usually look and feel. Do BSE to find any change from what is normal for you.

If you still menstruate, the best time to do BSE is 2 or 3 days after your period ends. These are the days when your breasts are least likely to be tender or swollen.

If you no longer menstruate, pick a certain day—such as the first day of each month—to remind yourself to do BSE.

If you are taking hormones, talk with your doctor about when to do BSE.

Here's what you should do to check for changes in your breasts.

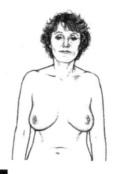

1 Stand in front of a mirror that is large enough for you to see your breasts clearly. Check each breast for anything unusual. Check the skin for puckering, dimpling, or scaliness. Look for a discharge from the nipples.

Do steps 2 and 3 to check for any change in the shape or contour of your breasts. As you do these steps, you should feel your chest muscles tighten.

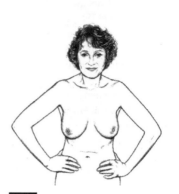

3 Next, press your hands firmly on your hips and bend slightly toward the mirror as you pull your shoulders and elbows forward.

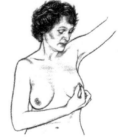

4 Gently squeeze each nipple and look for a discharge.

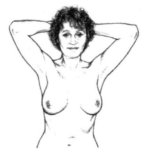

2 Watching closely in the mirror, clasp your hands behind your head and press your hands forward.

FIGURE **4-2** Technique for BSE. (From The National Cancer Institute.)

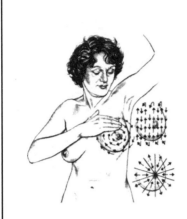

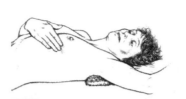

5 Raise one arm. Use the pads of the fingers of your other hand to check the breast and the surrounding area—firmly, carefully, and thoroughly. Some women like to use lotion or powder to help their fingers glide easily over the skin. Feel for any unusual lump or mass under the skin.

Feel the tissue by pressing your fingers in small, overlapping areas about the size of a dime. To be sure you cover your whole breast, take your time and follow a definite pattern: lines, circles, or wedges.

Some research suggests that many women do BSE more thoroughly when they use a pattern of up-and-down lines or strips. Other women feel more comfortable with another pattern. The important thing is to cover the whole breast and to pay special attention to the area between the breast and the underarm, including the under-arm itself. Check the area above the collarbone and all the way over to your shoulder.

Lines: Start in the underarm area and move your fingers downward little by little until they are below the breast. Then move your fingers slightly toward the middle and slowly move back up. Go up and down until you cover the whole area.

Circles: Beginning at the outer edge of your breast, move your fingers slowly around the whole breast in a circle. Move around the breast in smaller and smaller circles, gradually working toward the nipple. Don't forget to check the underarm and upper chest areas, too.

Wedges: Starting at the outer edge of the breast, move your fingers toward the nipple and back to the edge. Check your whole breast, covering one small wedge-shaped section at a time. Be sure to check the underarm area and the upper chest.

6 It's important to repeat step 5 while you are lying down. Lie flat on your back, with one arm over your head and a pillow or folded towel under the opposite shoulder. This position flattens the breast and makes it easier to check. Check each breast and the area around it very carefully using one of the patterns described above.

7 Some women repeat step 5 in the shower. Your fingers will glide easily over soapy skin, so you can concentrate on feeling for changes underneath.

If you notice a lump, a discharge, or any other change during the month—whether or not it is during BSE—contact your doctor.

FIGURE **4-2,** cont'd

including incomplete penetrance and etiologic heterogeneity, (6) risks of genetic testing including the potential for loss of insurance or employment and adverse psychosocial consequences for oneself and one's family, (7) options for prevention and surveillance and their limitations, and (8) assurance of confidentiality of test results and related information.[21] How would you judge this as a plan for the educational session?

4. A diagram for performing BSE may be found in Figure 4-2.[27] How would you use this diagram to teach low-income women?

5. Patients talk about "chemo brain"—a condition of difficulty with memory, attention, and new learning occurring after administration of chemotherapy, which may cause patients not to take oral chemotherapeutic agents. Is "chemo brain" real?

REFERENCES

1. Ansell D and others: A nurse-delivered intervention to reduce barriers to breast and cervical cancer screening in Chicago inner city clinics, *Pub Health Rep* 109:104-111, 1994.

2. Asbury N, Walshe A: Involving women with breast cancer in the development of a patient information leaflet for anticipatory nausea and vomiting, *Eur J Oncol Nurs* 9:33-43, 2005.

3. Breslow RA and others: Americans' knowledge of cancer risk and survival, *Prev Med* 26:170-177, 1997.

4. Bront JM, Fallsdown D, Iverson ML: The evolution of a breast health program for Plains Indian women, *Oncol Nurs Forum* 26:731-739, 1999.

5. Bruera E and others: The addition of an audiocassette recording of a consultation to written recommendations for patients with advanced cancer, *Cancer* 86:2420-2425, 1999.

6. Chalmers KI, Luker KA: Breast self-care practices in women with primary relatives with breast cancer, *J Adv Nurs* 23:1212-1220, 1996.

7. Chalmers K, Thomson K, Degner LF: Information, support and communication needs of women with a family history of breast cancer, *Cancer Nurs* 19:204-213, 1996.

8. Davis S, Stewart S, Bloom J: Increasing the accuracy of perceived breast cancer risk: results from a randomized trial with Cancer Information Service callers. *Prev Med* 39:64-73, 2004.

9. Davis TC and others: Knowledge and attitude on screening mammography among low-literate, low-income women, *Cancer* 78:1912-1920, 1996.

10. Deane KA, Degner LF: Determining the information needs of women after breast biopsy procedures, *AORN J* 65:767-776, 1997.

11 Erwin DO and others: Increasing mammography and breast self-examination in African American women using the Witness Project model, *J Cancer Educ* 11:210-215, 1996.

12. Fife BL: The measurement of meaning in illness, *Soc Sci Med* 40:1021-1028, 1995.

13. Fitch MI and others: Health promotion and early detection of cancer in older adults: assessing knowledge about cancer, *Oncol Nurs Forum* 24:1743-1748, 1997.

14. Flood AB and others: The importance of patient preference in the decision to screen for prostate cancer, *J Gen Intern Med* 11:342-349, 1996.

15. Gray RE and others: The information needs of well, long-term survivors of breast cancer, *Patient Educ Couns* 33:245-255, 1998.

16. Gregg J, Curry RH: Explanatory models for cancer among African-American women at two Atlanta neighborhood health centers: the implications for a cancer screening program, *Soc Sci Med* 39:519-526, 1994.

17. Hodge FS, Fredericks L, Rodriguez B: American Indian women's talking circle: a cervical screening and prevention project, *Cancer* 78(7 suppl):1592-1597, 1996.

18. Irwin E and others: Offering a choice between two adjuvant chemotherapy regimens: a pilot study to develop a decision aid for women with breast cancer, *Patient Educ Couns* 37:283-291, 1999.

19. Kash KM and others: Psychological counseling strategies for women at risk of breast cancer, *Monogr Natl Cancer Inst* 7:73-79, 1995.

20. Kash KM and others: Psychosocial aspects of cancer genetics: women at high risk for breast and ovarian cancer. *Semin Surg Oncol* 18:333-338, 2000.

21. Lerman C and others: What you don't know can hurt you: adverse psychologic effects in members of BRCA1-linked and BRCA2-linked families who decline genetic testing, *J Clin Oncol* 16:1650-1654, 1998.

22. Lethborg CE, Kissane DW: "It doesn't end on the last day of treatment": a psychoeductional intervention for women after adjuvant treatment for early stage breast cancer. *J Psychosoc Oncol* 21:25-41, 2003.

23. Marteau TM, Senior V, Sasieni P: Women's understanding of a "normal smear test result": experimental questionnaire based study, *BMJ* 322:526-528, 2001.

24. Miaskowski C and others: Randomized clinical trial of the effectiveness of a self-care intervention to improve cancer pain management. *J Clin Oncol* 22:1713-1720, 2004.

25. Neale J and others: An observational study of precolposcopy education sessions: what do women want to know? *Health Care Women Intl* 24:468-475, 2003.

26. Northouse LL, Peters-Golden H: Cancer and the family: strategies to assist spouses, *Semin Oncol Nurs* 9:74-82, 1993.

27. Pickett M, Barg FK, Lynch MP: Development of a home-based family caregiver cancer education program. *Hospice J* 15:19-39, 2001.

28. Redman BK: *Measurement tools in patient education,* ed 2, New York, 2003, Springer.

29. Sawka CA and others: Development of a patient decision aid for choice of surgical treatment for breast cancer. *Health Expectations* 1:23-36, 1998.

30. Sheridan-Leos N: Women's Health Loteria: a new cervical cancer education tool for Hispanic females, *Oncol Nurs Forum* 22:697-701, 1995.

31. Snyder LA and others: Development of the breast cancer education and risk assessment program, *Oncol Nurs Forum* 30:803-808, 2003.

32. Weinrich SP and others: Increasing prostate cancer screening in African American men with peer-educator and client-navigator interventions, *J Cancer Educ* 13:213-219, 1998.

33. West MD, Finney JW: Training in early cancer detection and anxiety in adolescent males: a preliminary report, *Dev Behav Pediatr* 17:98-99, 1996.

34. Yates P and others: A randomized controlled trial of a nurse-administered educational intervention for improving cancer pain management in ambulatory settings, *Patient Educ Couns* 53:227-237, 2004.

5

Cardiovascular and Pulmonary Patient Education

CARDIOVASCULAR PATIENT EDUCATION

CASE I

A phone survey of 751 patients with congestive heart failure (CHF) treated at hospitals, health plans, and cardiology physician group practices found self-reported education as described in Table 5-1. Only 14% of patients knew how to monitor their weight, monitored their weight regularly, and knew appropriate responses to deal with a weight increase on their own without consulting a physician or nurse. More than one fourth had not been taught which foods actually had a high salt content. The authors note that, although patient care guidelines and good patient education programs are available, they appear to be only moderately well applied. Why might this be?

Educational Approaches and Research Base

Approximately 58 million persons in the United States (20% of the total population) have one or more types of cardiovascular disease, which includes high blood pressure (BP), coronary heart disease, stroke, rheumatic fever or disease, or other forms of heart disease.[43] Reported educational programs in the cardiovascular area deal with topics that involve alteration of risk factors, including hypertension and hyperlipidemias, management of heart failure, decrease in time delay until treatment for acute myocardial infarction (AMI) and stroke, implementation of cardiac rehabilitation after AMI or cardiac surgery, regimen maintenance, and self-management of anticoagulation.

In the 1970s and 1980s several countries, including the United States, invested in large-scale clinical research trials designed to decrease cardiovascular risk factors—high BP, smoking, high blood cholesterol levels, excess weight, and lack of exercise—by facilitating adoption of health practices in entire communities. The interventions lasted 5 to 8 years and frequently used a theoretical framework based on principles of behavioral change. Interventions focused on changing the community environment, training indigenous leaders, educational self-help, and

TABLE 5-1 Participants' Self-Reported Education Received	% Yes*
Pathophysiology and treatment	
Explained what is wrong with your heart?	74.5
Explained why you sometimes feel tired, short of breath, or have swelling in your legs?	72.5
Explained how your medicines work and the benefits of taking the medicine?	82.2
Mean Percent Received	77.3
Lifestyle modifications and monitoring	
Told you not to use salt when you cook, not to add salt to your food after it is cooked?	85.5
Talked with you about which foods are high in salt and which are not?	73.8
Told you to avoid drinking alcohol?[†]	76.3[†]
Told you to avoid drinking large amounts of water or other fluids?	46.9
Told you to weigh yourself on a scale every morning and write down your weight?	57.9
Told you that you should get regular exercise, such as walking?	85.8
Mean Percent Received	70.8[†]
Medication compliance	
Encouraged you to use a pillbox to help you keep track of or organize your medicine?	52.4
Talked with you about techniques for remembering to take your medicine every day?	48.1
Asked whether you can afford your medicines?	29.0
Mean Percent Received	43.5
Prognosis and preferences for end-of-life care	
Talked with you about how your heart condition might affect how long you live?	37.5
Talked with you about living wills, durable power of attorney for health care, or other ways of writing down what you would want done?	42.6
Mean Percent Received	40.7
Mean overall education index score, range 0-13 (SD)	7.9 (3.0)

*Two patients did not answer this section, leaving 779 for analysis.
[†]The percentage shown is based on patients for whom alcohol counseling applies (468/613). The mean percent received excludes the alcohol item because this question was not applicable to all patients.
(From Baker DW, Brown J, Chan KS, Dracup KA, Keeler EB: A telephone survey to measure communication, education, self-management, and health status for patients with heart failure: the Improving Chronic Illness Core Evaluation (ICICE), *J Card Fail* 11:36-42, 2005.)

diffusion of the innovation through social networks in the community, in part to provide people with social support to maintain the initial action.

Multimedia campaigns were aimed at large audiences and were carefully segmented to influence individuals to change behavior by using clear, repetitive messages. The impact of these programs was modest, with improvement in behavioral risk factors but equivocal effects on biological risk factors such as BP and blood cholesterol levels. Effects on actual cardiovascular heart disease risk are yet to be shown.[56]

Although the popularity of large community studies has waned, community-based education is still used to decrease risk factors and patient delay of treatment and is very important for population subgroups that have not been reached successfully (e.g., ethnic minority groups, adults with low literacy levels, older women).

The National Cholesterol Education Program is a national campaign using mass media to promote lowering of the blood cholesterol distribution in the entire population. It has used two strategies: a patient-based or clinical approach and a population-based approach for those with hypercholesterolemia. The campaign cites as evidence of success the fact that from 1983 to 1995 the percentage of the public who had heard of high blood cholesterol rose from 77% to 93%, from 1986 to 1995 the proportion who knew that a desirable blood cholesterol level was below 200 mg/dl jumped from 16% to 69%, from 1983 to 1995 the percentage of U.S. adults who had ever had their cholesterol level checked climbed from 35% to 75%, and the percentage who knew their own levels increased from 3% to 49%.[15] In 1991 the National Heart Attack Alert Program was launched to educate health care providers, patients, and the general public about the importance of rapid and appropriate response to symptoms and signs of AMI.[19]

A review (not a meta-analysis) of 46 studies of cognitive, educational, and behavioral strategies to improve compliance with cardiovascular disease risk reduction found that successful strategies included signed agreements, self-efficacy enhancement, behavioral skill training, and telephone-mail contact. The comparative efficacy of these approaches was generally not tested.[12] A meta-analysis of 102 studies testing the effects of patient education and psychosocial support on blood pressure found statistically significant large treatment effects on knowledge and compliance and small to medium-sized statistically significant beneficial effects on blood pressure.[17] A meta-analysis of 37 studies of health education and stress management programs for patients with coronary heart disease found that these programs yielded a 34% decrease in mortality from cardiac disease, a 29% decrease in recurrence of AMI, and significant effects on BP, cholesterol, body weight, smoking behavior, physical exercise, and eating habits.[20] In addition, a meta-analysis[23] of randomized controlled trials of the addition of psychosocial treatments to traditional exercise-based cardiac rehabilitation regimens found that they decreased mortality and morbidity, psychological distress, and some biological risk factors, especially during the first 2 years after the intervention.[38]

Understanding patient delay in seeking care after symptoms of AMI or stroke has long been a high priority. Since the mid 1980s, several large-scale studies have demonstrated that thrombolytic therapy can significantly reduce mortality from AMI: the shorter the interval, the better the outcome. Yet over the past three decades, there has been little success in reducing delay time, including that for second AMIs.

The phenomenon of delay needs to be understood before education and counseling strategies to reduce delay can be designed. Approximately one third of patients do not report an abrupt onset of symptoms and frequently have difficulty identifying the time of onset. These patients may report vague symptoms or symptoms that wax and wane over time, sometimes disappearing completely. Knowledge of the symptoms of AMI does not ensure that a patient will recognize or acknowledge his or her own AMI symptoms and does not reduce delay in seeking health care.[18] Many subjects reported that they had expectations about the symptoms of heart disease that focused on location, intensity, associated symptoms, and quality. Expectations did not match the symptom experience of 74% of subjects, and these individuals delayed significantly longer before seeking treatment than did subjects whose expectations did match their experience. The longest phase is the time it takes individuals to interpret their symptoms as cardiac and decide to seek medical attention.[32]

Thus, despite widespread educational campaigns through public media, patient delay may not be affected because there is no uniform presenting syndrome for patients with AMI[32]; therefore, the educational content provided to patients may not be accurate for them. Although knowledge of chest pain as an important heart attack symptom is high and relatively uniform, knowledge of arm pain or numbness, shortness of breath, sweating, and other important symptoms is less common, especially among those of lower socioeconomic status and racial and ethnic minority groups. Risk factor status has not been found to be associated with knowledge of heart attack symptoms.[29] A number of instructional approaches have been suggested but as yet are untested, including the use of role model stories based on the real experiences of patients with heart attacks. The wall poster shown in Figure 5-1 provides a very specific protocol, which can also be made into a wallet card. Patients may not follow such instructions because they are made to feel foolish when their judgment about presenting themselves in emergency departments is questioned.

Zapka and others[63] find that a substantial portion of providers questioned the appropriateness of 911 use; some primary care physicians preferred that patients call them before 911, even though this approach frequently creates delays in treatment. Some physicians believed that telling patients about symptoms would stimulate their feeling these symptoms. Many nurses believed physicians were not well prepared to teach patients and at the same time were not supportive of nurses doing so.

Management of Cardiovascular Risk Factors

Although the importance of BP control in preventing cardiovascular disease and stroke is well established and there are effective ways of reducing it, estimates suggest that fewer than 30% of hypertensive patients in the United States have their BPs under control. Although knowledge is rarely sufficient for health behaviors, it clearly is an important prerequisite. Lack of knowledge of target systolic BP has been shown to be an independent predictor of poor BP control, especially important in an aging population because systolic BP rises with age. Yet hypertension patient education programs have been shown to be associated with significant reductions in both systolic and diastolic BP. The knowledge base of 2500 hypertension patients from a large health maintenance organization showed that more than 60% were not aware of systolic and diastolic BP targets to aim for. Approximately one half of all subjects with elevated systolic and diastolic BPs were not aware that these BP values were too high. Although most of the 2500 understood that hypertension increased the risk for development of stroke and heart attack, about half were aware that it increased the risk of heart failure and 40% that it increased the risk of kidney disease.[1]

Blood pressure control by home monitoring offers more frequent measurement in a familiar setting, avoiding "white coat" hypertension. This approach is also well studied. Cappuccio and colleagues[13] performed a meta-analysis of 18 randomized controlled trials of home monitoring and found it superior to standard BP monitoring in the health care system in achieving target BP levels. Home BP telemonitoring allows patients to take their BP, store the data, and then transmit data through a toll-free number over existing telephone lines to a network server provided by a telemonitoring service. The server generates BP reports and sends them to health care providers. These monitors do not allow individuals to adjust their readings, thereby giving health care providers more confidence in the home-collected BP data and thus in the resulting clinical decisions.[4]

Dyslipidemias involve alterations in plasma lipoproteins or their metabolism and are considered to be a major but modifiable risk factor for coronary heart disease. They may be manifested by an elevation of in serum levels of total cholesterol, low-density lipoprotein cholesterol (LDL-C), or triglycerides in conjunction with a low concentration of high-density lipoprotein cholesterol (HDL-C). It has been estimated that a quarter of the U.S. adult population requires aggressive lower-ing of LDL-C levels. Patient education by pharmacists improved the LDL/HDL ratio by 17.2%.[2]

Other risk factors such as obesity require dietary and exercise lifestyle changes, difficult for many to undertake. Oexmann and others[49] found a church-based approach among African-Americans to provide the structure and motivation to attain short-term reductions in weight, mean BP, and triglyceride levels. Lighten Up was developed in collaboration with members of the local faith community and consisted of a baseline health assessment, eight weekly educational sessions combining Bible study with a health message, a short-term health assessment at 11 weeks, and a long-term health assessment at 52 weeks. It was especially effective in those who attended six to eight sessions.

A cardiovascular nutrition educational approach tailored for individuals of limited literacy used food-picture cards showing low, medium, or high in fat, cholesterol, and sodium; a nutrition guide;

Chest Pain Can Be An Emergency

If you feel any of the following
- Chest pain or discomfort that is very bad and lasts longer than 15 minutes,
- Chest discomfort along with weakness, feeling sick to your stomach, feeling faint or dizzy, and sweating,
- Chest discomfort that feels like tightness, pressure, burning, or heaviness that lasts for about 15 minutes,
- Sudden shortness of breath with no other cause . . .

A Heart Attack can also feel like . . .
- A mild chest discomfort, that may go on and off even when you are at rest,
- Or it may feel like regular heartburn, or indigestion.
  - Note the time the chest discomfort starts.
  - If it feels like heartburn, take some antacid like TUMS, Mylanta, or whatever it is you usually take for heartburn.
  - Note how long your discomfort lasts.
  - IF THE "MILD CHEST DISCOMFORT" OR "HEARTBURN" LASTS FOR 15 MINUTES OR MORE,

ASK TO BE TAKEN TO THE EMERGENCY ROOM.
Have it checked out. Better safe than sorry.

If you already have prescription for nitroglycerin
- When the discomfort starts, sit down, and take 3 nitroglycerin one at a time - 5 minutes apart.
- IF AFTER THE THIRD ONE, THE PAIN OR DISCOMFORT IS STILL THERE (even if it's mild),

ASK TO BE TAKEN TO THE EMERGENCY ROOM.

DO NOT DRIVE YOURSELF TO THE HOSPITAL!
- If your community emergency number is not 911, the number to call is _____
- If your community does not have an emergency number, your driver's name and phone number are _____
  _____
- Your doctor's name and phone number are _____
  _____

- I will keep my EKG in my wallet.
- I will bring it with me every time I go to the hospital or doctor.

- I will call **The Professionals** at any time if I have questions about what to do in cases where I am unsure.

FIGURE **5-1** A sample wall poster/handout. (From Blank FSJ and others: Development of an ED teaching program aimed at reducing prehospital delays for patients with chest pain, *J Emerg Nurs* 24:316-319, 1998.)

video and audiotape series using a family culturally similar to the target group; worksheets; and four classes. The materials were formatted to minimize literacy demands. Participants were instructed to select, ignore, and rearrange the food cards according to preferences and eating patterns and to involve members in playing games with them such as guessing the level of fat in a particular food. Those who participated in this program showed significant improvements in BP and lipid profiles.[37]

Congestive Heart Failure Self-Management Education

This field of patient education and the dramatic results that can be attained have recently been discovered. CHF is the most common indication for hospital admission among older adults, with up to 40% being readmitted in 6 months, often because of inadequate self-management skills. Half of these rehospitalizations are believed to be preventable. Patients must feel confident to carry out instructions for the prescribed diet and medical management and to monitor weight and symptoms for worsening of their disease (weight gain, edema, orthopnea, and fatigue). Patients often have no idea what heart failure is and know only about heart attack and fat rather than sodium and fluids.

Intervention approaches shown to effectively prevent hospital readmission include case management, telemanagement, multidisciplinary teams, and nurse-run clinics. In all of these approaches, patient education and intensive follow-up are central. Some interventions are as minimal as sending packets of information and videotapes to a patient's home. Heidenrich and others[31] report results of a randomized controlled trial in which patients at home received a digital scale and an automatic BP cuff and were taught to use them. Each day the patient called a toll-free number and entered the BP, pulse, weight, and symptoms into a computerized voice answering system. A computer algorithm checked them with an acceptable range and, if the readings were outside this range or there were new symptoms, the computer paged a nurse who called the patient and faxed the results to the physician. In this intervention

patients received weekly educational mailings providing instruction on diet, exercise, and common therapies and a 10-minute call from the nurse discussing these topics. Intervention programs are often very cost-effective with an 8:1 return on investment.[59]

In another study a Web-based monitoring system included a medication compliance device that linked the patient's telephone line with an Internet-accessible database. The device prompted patients about a heart-healthy diet, physical activity, and medication taking and requested answers to questions about symptoms, BP, and weight. Medication-compliance data and answers to questions were recorded by the device and up-loaded daily to a central server. By use of a standard browser interface, clinicians were able to monitor the patients, provide advice, and update the treatment regimens. Pilot data showed better adherence to medications and daily BP and weight monitoring compared with usual care. All patients received an educational booklet describing CHF self-care.[3]

Others have sought ways to decrease skilled home visits while improving outcomes by avoiding costly rehospitalizations in these patients. In one telehealth program, families are instructed in the use of the home monitor. Every morning at a preset time the monitor prompts the patient in a clear audible voice and guides the patient in assessing weight, BP, heart rate, and oxygen saturation. The monitor then asks three subjective questions about increased edema, shortness of breath, or the use of extra pillows to sleep comfortably. These data are then transmitted by phone line or wireless pager to the central station located in the home care agency office and reviewed by a clinician who initiates any necessary follow-up including calling the patient for further assessment, calling the attending physician, coordinating medication adjustments, and if necessary making a visit. Patients and family also must learn that the monitor is not a life-saving device and that if there is a true cardiac emergency, they must contact 911. Before this program was implemented, the agency's 30-day hospital readmission rate for CHF was 38%; within 2 months of the program, the readmission rate dropped to 6%.

Thus, patient outcomes and satisfaction have dramatically improved and the home care agency has been able to maintain its financial viability in a limited prospective pay environment.[53]

Patients with CHF seem to need not only a structured program of education but also regular follow-up, in part because they must manage a complex treatment plan involving multiple medications and rigorous self-care practices and may also be dealing with other comorbid conditions. But a 1 hour one-on-one teaching session with a nurse educator compared with the standard discharge process found subjects randomized to receive the teaching session had fewer days hospitalized and fewer days to death in the follow-up period than did controls, and costs of care including the cost of the intervention were lower by $2823 per patient. The education session covered causes of intravascular volume overload in heart failure, mechanism of action of diuretic medications, role of dietary restriction of sodium and water intake, daily weight monitoring, and what to do if symptoms worsened.[36]

Others have designed transitional care programs for persons with CHF—a 3-month advance practice nurse (APN)–directed discharge planning and home follow-up protocol. APNs made daily visits while the patient was in the hospital, a home visit within 24 hours of discharge, weekly visits during the first month, and if the patient was rehospitalized went back to daily visits. All patient education was audiotaped and left for patients and caregivers to review. Although time to first readmission or death was longer in intervention patients and total costs lower, transitional care programs such as this have typically not been adopted because of lack of Medicare reimbursement.[47]

Finally, disease management programs include the education and systematic follow-up/monitoring described above but do so on a defined population of patients with the disease. Seventy-five percent of managed care plans indicated that they offer CHF disease-management programs In a study of one, significant reductions in hospitalizations, emergency department visits, and short-term skilled nursing facility stays were found with no significant changes in office visits. Total

claims costs in the intervention group were 10% less than in the control group with intervention costs included.[7]

CASE II

Data from more than 81,000 patient admissions for heart failure at 223 academic and nonacademic hospitals in the United States showed a 24% conformity to Joint Commission on Accreditation of Healthcare Organizations guidelines to supply the patient or caregiver with written instructions and guidance on specific aspects of postdischarge care such as activity level, diet and fluid, names of discharge medications, follow-up with health care provider, weight monitoring, and what to do if heart failure symptoms worsen. The gap between counseling and instructions and the standards was significantly greater at academic than at nonacademic centers. Of the four guidelines for standards for care of patients with heart failure, lack of discharge instruction was by far the worst.[24]

A) Are you surprised by these findings? B) What would you suggest to correct the problem?

Stroke

Stroke is the third leading cause of death and the leading cause of adult disability.[50] Stroke prevention and self-management patient education has been less common than has similar education for AMI. Statistics show that only 5% of patients seek treatment for stroke in less than 3 hours, symptoms are not recognized, and patients and family think nothing can be done, or that the situation is not an emergency.[16] As for AMI, knowledge of stroke symptoms is not associated with early presentation to the emergency department; neither is having had a prior stroke.[61]

Education has been shown to be important in three respects. Morrison and others[44] show significantly lower anxiety and depression among patients with acute strokes who were educated with a self-help workbook. Wiles and others[60] find that caregivers for persons with stroke needed information about coping with daily care activities of bathing and dressing; the significance of symptoms such as memory loss, swallowing difficulties, irritability, and depression; how these symptoms could be managed; and how long they might last. Finally, a decision aid can be used to assist patients with atrial fibrillation, and therefore an increased risk of stroke, to choose between warfarin and aspirin therapy for stroke prevention. Like hormone replacement therapy and benign prostatic hypertrophy, the relative values of the benefits and risks are a matter of patient choice.[39]

Advances in stroke rehabilitation have decreased severe disability and increased the number of disabled patients living at home supported by caregivers who often feel inadequately trained, poorly informed, and dissatisfied with the support available after discharge. A randomized controlled trial compared conventional support (information on stroke, consequences, prevention and management, goal setting for rehabilitation and discharge) with additional instruction for caregivers (common stroke-related problems and their prevention, pressure areas, continence, nutrition, positioning, gait facilitation, advice on benefits and local services, hands-on training in lifting and handling, mobility and transfers, continence, assistance with activities of daily living [ADL], and communication). Training started when patient rehabilitation needs had stabilized and discharge was contemplated. Caregivers received three to five 30- to 40-minute sessions and a follow-through session at home. Supplemental training was associated with better caregiver quality of life and psychological outcomes and lower costs over a year because of less hospitalization.[33]

Anticoagulation Self-Management Training

Long-term anticoagulation is used to reduce stroke risk in atrial fibrillation and in mechanical heart valve replacement; this therapy is also used to treat venous thromboembolism. Pharmacodynamic response to these medications is unpredictable, much of the intraindividual variability is unexplained, and they have a narrow therapeutic range. Traditionally, patients receiving anticoagulation therapy have been monitored in hospital-based clinics or in provider practices. Patient self-management of this therapy improves

anticoagulation control over these traditional practices, probably as a result of more frequent monitoring and dose adjustment, which results in fewer thromboembolic or bleeding events, potentially serious side effects of the treatment.[35] Development of portable coagulometers has made self-management possible.

Several studies have shown education separate from and sometimes in addition to self-management yields more time in the therapeutic range. Khan and others[35] showed that both of these forms of education had the desired effect; significant improvements in anticoagulation control were noted after just one educational session. Christensen and colleagues[14] found that self-managing patients were in the therapeutic range 76% of the time, in contrast to those in highly specialized anticoagulation clinics and using computer dosing in the target range 60% to 68% of the time. Menendez-Jandula and others[41] found that 4 hours of instruction for monitoring and self-adjustment of treatment dose, split between 2 days, provided better control than did an anticoagulation clinic with monthly measurement and control managed by hematologists. Major and minor complications were less common in the self-management group.

It is generally felt that patients must be carefully selected to self-manage this therapy. Some patients are highly motivated to self-manage because they are then free for other life commitments rather than remaining tied to a hospital clinic.[14] A study in the United Kingdom found that 76% of patients invited chose not to undertake self-management. Of unselected patients keen to undertake self-management, three fourths were able to complete training. Manual difficulties with the procedure and trouble obtaining sufficient capillary blood and placing the sample on the test strip were noted.[46] In the Menendez-Jandula study, 90% of patients had primary school education or were illiterate.[41] Adaptive teaching approaches included a simple card system to help patients select correct doses. In this study, 310 patients were trained in self-management, 10 patients could not be trained and were returned to conventional management, and 39 required some help from a caregiver.

Other Topics

Other areas of patient education include cardiac surgery and cardiac rehabilitation with well-developed educational models, new areas such as cardiopulmonary resuscitation (CPR) training for families, classes for those with mitral valve prolapse, and the continuing mystery about why people with symptoms of AMI (or stroke for that matter) do not heed or interpret them and seek help.

Patient education initiatives surrounding cardiac surgery are summarized in Table 5-2. The last part of that series, cardiac rehabilitation, has consistently been underenrolled, particularly by women. Although it has been shown to improve functional status, cardiac risk factor profiles, and psychosocial well-being to a similar extent in young and old patients, in the case of revascularization patients only a quarter of those eligible actually enroll in a cardiac rehabilitation program. Pasquali and others[51] have shown that a simple postdischarge patient education and referral intervention nearly doubled enrollment. Patients reported feeling overwhelmed with the variety of instructions concerning new medications, follow-up appointments and so forth at the time of discharge, and appreciated the additional information regarding cardiac rehabilitation being provided at a later date. They needed to know of the potential health benefits and specifically how to enroll in the program.

Most cardiac arrests among cardiac patients occur at home in the presence of the spouse. The perception of control related to a partner's cardiac disease is associated with enhanced emotional adjustment on the part of the spouse and recovery on the part of the patient; therefore, it is reasonable to expect that perceived control could be increased in spouses by teaching them to respond appropriately with CPR if the partner had a cardiac arrest. One-person CPR was taught in small groups. Perceived control was unchanged in the control group but increased significantly in those taught CPR along with risk factor information or along with social support about the emotional issues raised by learning CPR.[45] One study has shown that CPR can be effectively taught through videotape self-instruction in the home, with skills being practiced during the showing, like an exercise video. Cardboard mannikins can be used both for the video and for practice. Training may be accomplished without an instructor in one eighth the time of traditional CPR instruction.[11]

Mitral valve prolapse (MVP) has a reported prevalence from 4% to 18% and is one of the most common congenital heart diseases, affecting millions of people. Many of those affected have arrhythmias, chest pain, shortness of breath, or dizziness with postural changes, all frightening symptoms that are interpreted to indicate that something is terribly wrong. Although most persons with this syndrome have a benign prognosis and rarely require valve replacement, MVP is rarely explained to them and information regarding self-care measures is infrequently provided. Many cities in the United States now have MVP support groups in which this information is provided.[54] MVP is a perfect example of a patient education need to which the formal health system does not respond; although it is usually benign, patients need help in making sense of the symptoms and their meaning.

PULMONARY PATIENT EDUCATION

Chronic Obstructive Pulmonary Disease

Chronic obstructive pulmonary disease (COPD) is the fourth leading cause of death in the United States, its incidence continuing to rise. This diagnosis encompasses chronic bronchitis, emphysema, asthmatic bronchitis, and bronchiectasis and is characterized by airflow obstruction and frequently by bronchial hyperreactivity in response to inhaled irritants such as tobacco smoke and dust. COPD is characterized by a significant and progressive reduction in expiratory airflow developing insidiously over many years. The National Lung Health Education Program is aimed at preventing premature morbidity and mortality from COPD by identifying the 15% to 20% of smokers in whom COPD will develop and patients with respiratory symptoms in whom airflow obstruction is just beginning to develop.[10]

Because of the role of cigarette smoking in causing the disease, persons with COPD have

TABLE 5-2	**Summary of Patient Education Initiatives**
Initiative	**Comments**
Information pack	Sent when patient placed on waiting list for surgery. Detailed information is given: • Preparing for your heart operation—provides information about the structure and function of the heart, different heart diseases, types of surgery, preparation for surgery, postoperative pain management and recovery, postoperative education, discharge from hospital, and rehabilitation • Inpatient information—including patients' rights regarding consent to operation
Presurgery preparation day	Attendance is advised, although patients who are unable to attend receive information packs. The day lasts about 4 hours with a break for lunch and is run by the cardiac liaison nurse. Topics covered: • Management of waiting lists • How the heart works • Types of heart operation • Preoperative and postoperative care • Discharge from hospital • Two videos are shown: *Intensive care—Your recovery after surgery* and *Life after heart surgery*
Preadmission clinic	The preadmission clinic is available for patients with a date for surgery. They can attend up to 1 month before their date of surgery. Attendance is compulsory for suitable patients. The morning component of the clinic is educational and the afternoon is spend completing tests and assessments. The clinic nurse gives patients an introductory talk on heart disease and an explanation of the operative procedure. A current patient talks about what the experience really feels like. An intensive treatment unit nurse speaks on immediate postoperative recovery, a physiotherapist speaks about postoperative mobility, and an occupational therapist speaks about resuming activities after surgery. In the afternoon, patients attend to the paperwork of the admission process and their consent to operative treatment is obtained and documented. The clinic nurse might quote the average risk of operative complications, but this information is rarely requested.
Postoperative education	While the patient is in hospital, she or he is encouraged to attend a series of ward teaching sessions held in the afternoons. They cover physiotherapy, pharmacy, diet, nursing, and occupational therapy
Cardiac rehabilitation	Patients are advised to attend a class 6 weeks after surgery covering all aspects of rehabilitation including exercise, stress reduction, etc

From Beresford N, Seymour L, Vincent C, Moat N: Risks of elective cardiac surgery: what do patients want to know? *Heart* 86:626-631, 2001. Reproduced with permission from the BMJ Publishing Group.

often been stigmatized with fatalistic attitudes regarding its control.[10] Recently, however, self-management (SM) education programs have been tested separately or in conjunction with pulmonary rehabilitation programs. The education program should enable persons with COPD to analyze the degree of their airflow limitation continuously at home, to check the efficiency of their medical treatment, and to change their drug regimen with respect to the actual degree of airflow limitation on their own, with clear-cut guidelines for emergency medical care. In contrast to asthma, the site of airflow limitation from COPD may be located in the peripheral airways so that regular monitoring of the peak expiratory flow (PEF) rate has been thought to be inaccurate. Others find that in combination with monitoring of cough, dyspnea, and the amount and color of sputum, the PEF rate is helpful.[62]

There are now a number of trials of varying degrees of rigor, testing patient education for this group, usually provided in outpatient settings with small groups of patients. Besides obtaining skills in monitoring respiratory function and altering medication, long-term oxygen therapy should be included for those with more severe disease. Although generally less successful than asthma education, presumably because of the high reversibility of symptoms and airflow limitations in asthma,[62] COPD SM education is moving beyond the experimental.

In a randomized controlled trial (RCT), Gallefoss[25] found that in patients with mild to moderate COPD a 4-hour educational intervention followed by individual SM sessions showed a decreased need for physician visits, a dramatic decrease in the need for reliever medication, and a decreased cost of care at 12-month follow-up. Notably, at the final educational session, the patient's understanding of his or her personal treatment plan was tested. Because the effects of full pulmonary rehabilitation programs frequently deteriorate quickly after the program ends, Gallefoss correctly raises the question of which patients need education and rehabilitation and which only education.

Finnerty and others[21] provided a 6-week program of education (2 hours weekly) and exercise (1 hour weekly) and found a significantly improved quality of life in patients with moderate to severe COPD in comparison with a control group, with the benefit still evident after 24 weeks. Bourbeau and others[9] also performed an RCT (although not blinded) of SM education with weekly health professional follow-up visits by health professionals for 2 months. Not only were hospitalizations for exacerbations of COPD decreased by 40% in the intervention as compared with the usual-care group, admissions for other health problems and emergency department visits were also considerably decreased, of greater magnitude than that reported in RCTs of pulmonary rehabilitation programs. This patient education program included skill-oriented, self-help workbook modules in inhalation technique, plan of action, breathing and coughing techniques, energy conservation and relaxation, preventing and controlling symptoms through inhalation techniques, healthy lifestyle, leisure and traveling, and home exercise.

An example of a well-designed pulmonary rehabilitation program for persons with COPD has been reported by Scherer, Schmiedler, and Shimmel.[52] Patients had 1-hour classes three times a week for 12 weeks with education in self-care, nutrition, stress management, and anxiety control; retraining in breathing techniques and dyspnea control; and work simplification followed by training and workout sessions. Because these patients often lack confidence in their ability to avoid breathing difficulty, it is important to build in techniques to increase patient self-efficacy—performance accomplishments, vicarious experience in watching others, verbal persuasion, and teaching control of emotional and physical arousal states. Community outings and active practice of pacing and energy conservation techniques into activities are important. Patients with higher self-efficacy showed a significant increase in activity. Pulmonary rehabilitation has also been reported as part of short-stay inpatient services.

Sometimes educational programs are focused on a particular symptom of COPD, particularly dyspnea. Two very different programs provide examples of how this may be accomplished. Stulberg and others[58] developed a dyspnea SM educational program with supervised exercise for persons with moderate to severe COPD, in four sessions over 8 weeks. The program focused on identification of each person's trigger for and understanding of dyspnea, medications, breathing retraining, distraction, and relaxation. Participants were instructed to walk at least four times per week for a minimum of 20 minutes at a pace sufficient to make them feel they could not have gone farther. Some received additional exposure to exercise-induced dyspnea with four nurse-coached treadmill exercise sessions for 30 minutes every other week for 8 weeks. There was a dose-dependent improvement in dyspnea with an increasing number of supervised exercise sessions.

In contrast, Nguyen and others[48] describe a dyspnea SM program delivered through the Internet for people with COPD, important because patients already short of breath have difficulty getting to an on-site class. Dyspnea with activities of daily living and self-efficacy for managing the symptom showed significant improvements in the intervention group with more modest changes in the overall sample. E-diaries, interactive group education with live chats, an individualized exercise plan negotiated by e-mail with each patient, patient-montored PEF rate, and forced expiratory volume were uploaded directly through phone lines to a central server and monitored by caregivers.

Clearly, SM education for COPD is poised to provide additional positive outcomes to patients.

Adults with Asthma

Morbidity and mortality from asthma have increased over the past decade despite improved understanding and advances in medical thera-peutics. Thirteen million people in the United States have this disease, which is characterized by episodic symptoms, variable airflow obstruc-tion and airway hyperresponsiveness, and inflam-mation. Asthma is the most common chronic disease of childhood, affecting one in 10 children. Among low-income families, many of whom have no health insurance, children with asthma have twice the odds of school failure as do those without the disease.[42] Childhood asthma is addressed in Chapter 7.

When asthma is managed appropriately, hospitalization is rarely required. Yet 43% of its economic impact is related to use of emergency services and hospitals, presumably resulting from failure of patients to effectively use preventive treatment. Adherence to preventive regimens does not improve with the severity of asthma. Table 5-3 and Box 5-1 describe the structure of asthma education as delivered in an office setting and asthma self-management plans for adults and children.[57] A version of this plan should be carried in the patient's wallet. Note that the plans integrate changes in PEF rate measurements (which can detect airway obstruction before symp-toms occur) or symptoms with written directions to introduce or increase therapy.

The highest level of lung function a patient is able to achieve after 1 to 2 weeks of aggressive therapy is the personal best for that patient and is used as a standard. This value should be re-assessed annually in adults and periodically in children. Asthma episodes rarely occur without warning; the symptoms patients experience at different degrees of falling from the personal best vary widely from patient to patient, but generally are consistent for each patient.[23] Identification and avoidance of triggers are also part of the plan; grasses, dust, temperature change, smoke, pets, cockroaches, upper respiratory infections, and exercise are common ones. Directions for use of a peak flow meter are shown in Box 5-2. Because studies have shown variable accuracy in PEF rate readings, patient technique should be checked at each clinic visit with retraining as needed if the technique has deteriorated.[26]

Each asthma plan must be individualized, taking into account the patient's personal best peak flow number and asthma signs and symp-toms. Behavioral goals of an asthma plan are early recognition of a change in the state of asthma stability that leads to early intervention for an exacerbation and sufficient confidence in the ability for self-management.

Because many classes of asthma medica-tions are available in metered dose-inhalers (MDI), learning the proper technique for self-administration is important. Only 20% to 40% of patients with asthma use the MDI correctly.

TABLE 5-3	**Essentials of Office Education for Patients with Asthma**	
Questions to Ask	**Educational Information in Easy-to-Understand Format**	**Skills to Teach the Patient and Have Demonstrated to Prove Proficiency**
First Office Visit		
What does having asthma mean to you?	Basic asthma facts	Inhalers and spacers (see patient information handout)
What medicines have you taken for your asthma and did they help?	Chronic lung disease	Introduce self-management plan (see Boxes 6-2 and 6-3)
What do you expect from asthma treatment?	Role of airways	Symptom monitoring
What do you want to accomplish with this visit?	Inflammation	Introduce use of peak flow monitoring if time permits (see patient information handout, Box 6-4)
Do you have any other questions for me today?	Role of bronchoconstriction	
	Intermittent airway narrowing	
	Asthma medications	
	Anti-inflammatory agents	
	Rescue medications: short-acting bronchodilators to relax smooth muscles	
	Bring list of all medicines and frequency of use to all appointments	
	Supply patient with office and hospital telephone numbers for advice	
Second Office Visit (2 to 4 Weeks after the First Visit or Sooner, as Needed)		
What medications are you taking and how often?	Use two types of medication	Self-management plan: Incorporate symptoms and peak flow monitoring
What problems have you had using your medications?	Reminder to bring peak flow meter and inhalers to all visits	Review goals
Show me how you use your inhalers.	Role of environmental control	Adjust peak flow monitoring as needed
Show me how you use your peak flow meter (if provided at first visit).	Allergens	Instruct patient in use of peak flow daily record and the need to bring meter and records to all visits (see Box 6-4)
	Irritants	Correct inhaler and spacer technique (patient should demonstrate proficiency at every visit)

From Stoloff SW, Janson S: Providing asthma education in primary care practice, *Am Fam Physician* 56:117-126, 1997.

TABLE 5-3	**Essentials of Office Education for Patients with Asthma—cont'd**	
Questions to Ask	**Educational Information in Easy-to-Understand Format**	**Skills to Teach the Patient and Have Demonstrated to Prove Proficiency**
All Subsequent Visits		

Ask all questions asked in previous visits
Ask if goals of therapy are being met
Ask patient, "What questions do you have about the self-management plan? Are you using it?"
Ask patient, "Do you have any new concerns about the therapy or your medications?"
	Review role of medications
	  Anti-inflammatory
	  Bronchodilators
	Review environmental control measures
	Review peak flow meter results in daily record, as needed
		Patient demonstrates technique in using inhaler, spacer, and peak flow meter
		Review and change self-management plan to meet goals of therapy

---

Box 5-1	*Self-Management Plan for the Treatment of Asthma*

Asthma is a disease of the airways in the lungs. The disease causes the airways to become inflamed, and this results in swelling and blockage. This makes it more difficult for you to breathe. Some simple steps can help you improve the management of your asthma. First, it's helpful to identify factors that trigger asthma episodes. You can then try to avoid the asthma triggers you and your doctor have identified. Keeping a record of your asthma symptoms and medications, and tracking your peak expiratory flow rate (PEFR), will also help you and your doctor manage your asthma. Use your peak expiratory flow meter every morning, or more often if needed, to measure the amount of airway blockage you have. Keep a daily record of the rates to show your doctor. Always use your peak flow meter at least once or twice a week. The morning rate is the best indicator of airway blockage. Be sure to write down your results. Use your peak flow meter more often if you notice decreasing flow rates or if you have symptoms of asthma or an upper respiratory infection (cough, wheeze, or chest tightness). When the PEFR results are falling, use the meter and write down the results at least twice a day, every day, so you can show them to your doctor.

First, you need to find out your "personal best" PEFR; your doctor will tell you how. The following explains how to manage your asthma according to your symptoms and your PEFR score:

A. If you don't have any symptoms that affect your work and play (no cough, no wheeze, no chest tightness) and your PEFR is greater than 80% to 85% of your personal best:
  Continue your normal maintenance dose schedule of medications:
  — Inhaled steroids, leukotriene modifiers (Accolate, Zyflo), cromolyn (Intal), or nedocromil (Tilade)
  — Oral theophylline

Continued

Box 5-1	*Self-Management Plan for the Treatment of Asthma—*cont'd

B. If you have symptoms (such as coughing, wheezing, chest tightness, waking at night with cough) and/or your PEFR is less than 80% of your usual results:

Use an inhaled bronchodilator. Take one puff and wait 1 to 2 minutes; then take another puff. You may take a third or fourth puff after waiting an additional 1 to 2 minutes between each puff. To determine the need for additional puffs, use the peak flow meter to check your PEFR. Use the best of three PEFR measurements. You may take more albuterol every hour to every 4 to 6 hours, depending on your PEFR results.

Double the dose of inhaled corticosteroid medication and take it more often, up to four times a day. (The maximum dosage for cromolyn and nedocromil is two puffs four times a day, unless your doctor tells you otherwise.) Don't take more than the following dosages of inhaled corticosteroids:

Beclomethasone (Beclovent, Vanceril), 20 puffs a day
Triamcinolone (Azmacort), 16 puffs a day
Flunisolide (AeroBid), 8 puffs a day
Budesonide (Pulmicort), 4 puffs a day
Fluticasone (Flovent), 800 to 1600 µg a day

Keep taking the increased dose until your PEFR is 80% (or better) of your personal best PEFR. Keep taking the increased dose for the same number of days it took you to get back to this PEFR level.

Reminder: Always be sure your technique of using the metered-dose inhaler is correct; if you aren't sure, call or visit your doctor.

C. If your symptoms are still getting worse even though you are following the above recommendations and/or if your PEFR is 60% or less of your personal best, start taking oral prednisone in the dosage prescribed by your doctor and call your doctor's office.

D. If your PEFR is 50% or less of your personal best, or if your PEFR is less than 150 to 200 liters per minute:

Call your doctor's office right away and go directly to the office or to the hospital emergency department, as directed.

Doctor's office telephone: _____
Hospital emergency department telephone:

_____

If you have any questions about this information or if you are having difficulty with your medicines or with the peak-flow meter, ask your doctor for information and help.

From Stoloff SW, Janson S: Providing asthma education in primary care practice, *Am Fam Physician* 56:117-126, 1997.

Box 5-2	*Correct Use of a Peak Flow Meter*

INSTRUCTIONS: To ensure that your peak flow measurements are correct, you must use the peak flow meter correctly. If you have difficulty with these directions or if you have any questions about using a peak flow monitor, please be sure to talk with your doctor.

1. Stand up.
2. Move the indicator on the peak flow meter to the bottom of the numbered scale.
3. Breathe out all your air and then take as deep a breath as you can (fill your lungs with air).
4. Put the mouthpiece of the meter in your mouth and close your lips around it.
5. Blow out as hard and as fast as you can.
6. Repeat steps 2 to 5 two more times (for a total of three times).
7. Write down the highest of the three numbers in your asthma record book.

From Stoloff SW, Janson S: Providing asthma education in primary care practice, *Am Fam Physician* 56:117-126, 1997.

Correct steps are the following: (1) take the cap off, (2) shake the MDI, (3) exhale to residual volume or functional residual capacity, (4) activate the inhaler with or slightly after the onset of inhalation, (5) take a steady deep inspiration, (6) hold breath for 10 seconds or as long as possible, (7) wait at least a minute before the next puff.[55] Individual products may have different directions.

Patients require frequent reinforcement of their self-management. The most common and important factor associated with a fatal outcome has been inability of the patient to recognize the severity of the attack. And it is patients who have the most severe asthma, with the greatest degree of bronchial hyperresponsiveness, who have the worst perception of the severity of airflow obstruction. These patients should be targeted for aggressive education and follow-up.[22] Indigent asthmatic patients who frequently use the emergency department as their primary source of care do respond well to repetitive education and follow-up, including removal of barriers to self-care, with significant decreases in the number of hospitalizations.[27,34]

Mortality from asthma is particularly high among racial and ethnic minorities compared with whites. In comparison with other patient groups, adults with asthma who have less education and lower income are likely to receive care that has less continuity and is less intensive after hospital discharge. These patients also have worse health and lower levels of physical and pulmonary function.[30]

Education about asthma and SM of asthma are now key recommendations of asthma management guidelines. A Cochrane systematic review[36] of RCTs involving 6090 participants found that asthma SM education that consists of information, self-monitoring, regular medical review, and a written action plan is effective and leads to a reduction in hospitalization and emergency department visits for asthma, unscheduled physician visits, days lost from work, episodes of nocturnal asthma, indirect cost, and an improvement in quality of life and in PEF. The effects were large enough to be of both clinical and statistical significance.[28]

In the six studies that compared these interventions, SM using a written action plan based on the PEF was found to be equivalent to SM using a symptoms-based written action plan. The PEF approach requires adjustment of medication on the basis of the best of three measurements morning and night. Compliance with PEF monitoring in the long term is poor, and some patients are poor perceivers of their symptoms.[28]

Markson and others[40] found that 30% of patients with asthma were dissatisfied with their current treatment, higher in those with a larger number of asthma control problems. The odds of treatment dissatisfaction were eight times higher among patients who reported uncertainty about the efficacy of their asthma medications or their ability to take the medication as directed than those without these disease management problems. It should be possible to identify regimens that patients believe will control their disease and that they can follow as directed by their providers.

SUMMARY

The most structured areas of cardiovascular patient education are reduction of risk factors, management of congestive heart failure, anticoagulation SM, and cardiac and stroke rehabilitation.

Pulmonary patient education continues for adults with asthma, with COPD patient education building on the asthma experience and demonstrating some significant successes. As with all chronic diseases, medical management and use of patient education toward important outcomes continue to fall significantly short of guidelines.

REFERENCES

1. Alexander M and others: Patient knowledge and awareness of hypertension is suboptimal: results from a large health maintenance organization, *J Clin Hypertens* 5:254-260, 2003.

2. Ali F and others: The effect of pharmacist intervention and patient education on lipid-lowering medication compliance and plasma cholesterol levels, *Can J Clin Pharmacol* 10:101-106, 2003.

3. Artinian NT and others: Pilot study of a Web-based compliance monitoring device for patients with congestive heart failure, *Heart Lung* 32:226-233, 2003.

4. Artinian NT and others: What you need to know about home blood pressure telemonitoring: but may not know to ask, *Home Healthcare Nurse* 22:680-686, 2004.

5. Baker DW and others: A telephone survey to measure communication, education, self-management, and health status for patients with heart failure: The Improving Chronic Illness Care Evaluation (ICICE), *J Card Failure* 11:36-42, 2005.

6. Beresford N and others: Risks of elective cardiac surgery: what do patients want to know? *Heart* 86:626-631, 2001.

7. Berg GD, Wadhwa S, Johnson AE: A matched-cohort study of health services utilization and financial outcomes for a heart failure disease-management program in elderly patients, *J Am Geriatr Soc* 52:1655-1661, 2004.

8. Blank FSJ and others: Development of an ED teaching program aimed at reducing prehospital delays for patients with chest pain, *J Emerg Nurs* 24:316-319, 1998.

9. Bourbeau J and others: Reduction of hospital utilization in patients with chronic obstructive pulmonary disease: a disease-specific self-management intervention, *Arch Int Med* 163:585-591, 2003.

10. Boyle AH, Waters HF: COPD: focus on prevention: Recommendations of the National Lung Health Education Program, *Heart Lung* 29:446-449, 2000.

11. Braslow A and others: CPR training without an instructor: development and evaluation of a video self-instructional system for effective performance of cardio-pulmonary resuscitation, *Resuscitation* 34:207-220, 1997.

12. Burke LE, Dunbar-Jacob JM, Hill MN: Compliance with cardiovascular disease prevention strategies: a review of the research, *Ann Behav Med* 19:239-263, 1997.

13. Cappuccio FP and others: Blood pressure control by home monitoring: meta-analysis of randomised trials, *BMJ* 329:145-148, 2004.

14. Christensen TD and others: Mechanical heart valve patients can manage oral anticoagulant therapy themselves, *Eur J Cardiothoracic Surg* 23:292-298, 2003.

15. Cleeman JI, L'enfant C: The National Cholesterol Education Program, *JAMA* 280:2099-2104, 1998.

16. Daley S and others: Education to improve stroke awareness and emergent response, *J Neurosci Nurs* 29:393-396, 1997.

17. Devine EC, Reifschneider E: A meta-analysis of the effects of psychoeducational care in adults with hypertension, *Nurs Res* 44:237-245, 1995.

18. Dracup K and others: Causes of delay in seeking treatment for heart attack symptoms, *Soc Sci Med* 40:379-392, 1995.

19. Dracup K and others: The physician's role in minimizing prehospital delay in patients at high risk for acute myocardial infarction: recommendations from the National Heart Attack Alert Program, *Ann Intern Med* 12:45-51, 1997.

20. Dusseldorf E and others: A meta-analysis of psychoeducational programs for coronary heart disease patients, *Health Psychol* 18:506-519, 1999.

21. Finnerty JP and others: The effectiveness of outpatient pulmonary rehabilitation in chronic disease, *Chest* 119:1705-1710, 2001.

22. Fishwick D, D'Souza WD, Beasley R: The asthma self-management plan system of care: what does it mean, how is it done, does it work, what models are available, what do patients want and who needs it? *Patient Educ Couns* 32:S21-S33, 1997.

23. Flaum M, Lang CL, Tinkelman D: Take control of high-cost asthma, *J Asthma* 34:5-14, 1997.

24. Fonarow GC, Yancy CW, Heywood JT: Adherence to heart failure quality-of-care indicators in US hospitals, *Arch Intern Med* 165:1469-1477, 2005.

25. Gallefoss F: The effects of patient education in COPD in a 1-year follow-up randomised, controlled trial, *Patient Educ Couns* 52:259-266, 2004.

26. Gannon PFG and others: The effect of patient technique on the accuracy of self-recorded peak expiratory flow, *Eur Respir J* 14:28-31, 1999.

27. George MR and others: A comprehensive educational program improves clinical outcome measures in inner-city patients with asthma, *Arch Intern Med* 159:1710-1716, 1999.

28. Gibson PG, Ram FSF, Powell H: Asthma education, *Respir Med* 97:1036-1044, 2003.

29. Goff DC and others: Knowledge of heart attack symptoms in a population survey in the United States, *Arch Intern Med* 158:2329-2338, 1998.

30. Haas JS and others: The impact of socioeconomic status on the intensity of ambulatory treatment and health outcomes after hospital discharge for adults with asthma, *J Gen Intern Med* 9:121-126, 1994.

31. Heidenrich PA, Ruggerio CM, Massio BM: Effect of a home monitoring system on hospitalization resource use for patients with heart failure, *Am Heart J* 138:633-640, 1999.

32. Johnson JA, King KB: Influence of expectations about symptoms on delay in seeking treatment during a myocardial infarction, *Am J Crit Care* 4:29-35, 1995.

33. Kalra L and others: Training care givers of stroke patients: randomised controlled trial, *BMJ* 328:1099-1101, 2004.

34. Kelso TM and others: Educational and long-term therapeutic intervention in the ED: effect on outcomes in adult indigent minority asthmatics, *Am J Emerg Med* 13:632-637, 1995.

35. Khan TI and others: The value of education and self-monitoring in the management of warfarin therapy in older patients with unstable control of anticoagulation, *Br J Haematol* 126:557-564, 2004.

36. Koelling TM and others: Discharge education improves clinical outcomes in patients with chronic heart failure, *Circulation* 111:179-185, 2005.

37. Kumanyika SK and others: Outcomes of a cardio-vascular nutrition counseling program in African-

Americans with elevated blood pressure or cholesterol level, *J Am Diet Assoc* 99:1380-1388, 1391, 1999.

38. Linden W, Stossel C, Maurice J: Psychosocial interventions for patients with coronary artery disease, *Arch Intern Med* 156:745-752, 1996.

39. Man-Son-Hing M and others: A patient decision aid regarding antibiotic therapy for stroke prevention in atrial thrombotic therapy for stroke prevention in atrial fibrillation, *JAMA* 282:737-743, 1999.

40. Markson LE and others: Insight into patient dissatisfaction with asthma treatment, *Arch Intern Med* 161:379-384, 2001.

41. Menendez-Jandula B and others: Comparing self-management of oral anticoagulant therapy with clinic management, *Ann Intern Med* 142:1-10, 2005.

42. Meurer JR and others: The Awesome Asthma School Days program: educating children, inspiring a community, *J Sch Health* 69:63-68, 1999.

43. Missed opportunities in preventive counseling for cardiovascular disease—U.S. 1995, *MMWR Morb Mortal Wkly Rep* 47:91-95, 1998.

44. Morrison VL and others: Improving emotional outcomes following acute stroke: a preliminary evaluation of a workbook-based intervention, *Scot Med J* 43:52-53, 1998.

45. Moser DK, Dracup K: Impact of cardiopulmonary resuscitation training on perceived control in spouses of recovering cardiac patients, *Res Nurs Health* 23:270-278, 2000.

46. Murray E and others: Training for patients in a randomised controlled trial of self management of warfarin treatment, *BMJ* 328:437-438, 2004.

47. Naylor MD and others: Transitional care of older adults hospitalized with heart failure: a randomized, controlled trial, *J Am Geriatr Soc* 52:675-684, 2004.

48. Nguyen H and others: Is Internet-based support for dyspnea self-management in patients with chronic obstructive pulmonary disease possible? Results of a pilot study, *Heart Lung* 34:51-62, 2005.

49. Oexmann MJ and others: Short-term impact of a church-based approach to lifestyle change on cardiovascular risk in African-Americans, *Ethn Dis* 10:17-23, 2000.

50. Pancioli AM and others: Public perception of stroke warning signs and knowledge of potential risk factors, *JAMA* 279:1288-1292, 1998.

51. Pasquali SK and others: Testing an intervention to increase cardiac rehabilitation enrollment after coronary artery bypass grafting, *Am J Cardiol* 88:1415-1416, 2001.

52. Scherer YK, Schmiedler LE, Shimmel S: The effects of education alone and in combination with pulmonary rehabilitation on self-efficacy in patients with COPD, *Rehab Nurs* 23:71-77, 1998.

53. Schneider NM: Managing congestive heart failure using home telehealth, *Home Healthcare Nurse* 22:719-722, 2004.

54. Scordo KAB: Factors associated with participation in a mitral valve prolapse support group, *Heart Lung* 30:128-137, 2001.

55. Shresta M and others: Metered-dose inhaler technique of patients in an urban ED: prevalence of incorrect technique and attempt at education, *Am J Emerg Med* 14:380-384, 1996.

56. Simons-Morton DG, Cutler JA: Cardiovascular disease prevention research at the National Heart, Lung and Blood Institute, *Am J Prev Med* 14:317-330, 1998.

57. Stoloff SW, Janson S: Providing asthma education in primary care practice, *Am Fam Physician* 56:117-126, 1997.

58. Stulbarg MS and others: Exercise training improves outcomes of a dyspnea self-management program, *J Cardiopul Rehabil* 22:109-121, 2002.

59. Study: CHF education more than pays for itself, *Health Benchmarks* 4:144-146, 1997.

60. Wiles R and others: Providing appropriate information to patients and carers following stroke, *J Adv Nurs* 28:794-801, 1998.

61. Williams LS and others: Stroke patients' knowledge of stroke, *Stroke* 28:912-915, 1997

62. Worth H, Dhein Y: Does patient education modify behaviour in the management of COPD? *Patient Educ Couns* 52:267-270, 2004.

63. Zapka J and others: Health providers' perspectives on patient delay for seeking care for symptoms of acute myocardial infarction, *Health Educ Behav* 26:714-733, 1999.

6

Diabetes Self-Management Education

CASE

You are teaching a diabetes education class to a dozen adults in the classroom of an inner city hospital. All have type II diabetes, diagnosed from 1 month to 20 years ago. Each has been seen individually before class and will be seen in an individual session 6 weeks after the class to attend to their special needs and goals. The class meets for three 3-hour sessions and has the following goals.

In addition to learning what diabetes is, you will learn to check your blood sugar; eat well while staying on plan; exercise for fun, fitness, and health; relax and reduce stress; take your medications/insulin properly; share feelings and anxieties about diabetes; recognize when blood sugar is high or low and what to do about it; prevent foot problems; maintain good health habits; and prevent and manage sick days.[5]

All teaching materials are included in a booklet given to participants. Class time is used for presentation of information included in the booklet, in an easy give-and-take discussion, using drawings (such as relationship between blood glucose, insulin levels and meals), case examples volunteered by participants, and a video on emotional reactions to and coping

with diabetes. After each major concept such as what is diabetes, long-term effects of high blood sugar, regulating the diabetes, the basics of eating, monitoring the diabetes, physical activity/exercise, and diabetes medications, there are a series of questions requiring participants to recall key information.

There is clearly an empowering tone to the classes, with an emphasis that 90% of diabetes care is what the participant does, and these classes will educate him or her to make choices toward a goal. Participants are told that they can control their blood sugar by what and how much they eat, and this is very powerful. Miniprotocols are used to address common problems, for example, what should you do when your blood sugar is high? (1) can you spot the cause? (good exercise, medication, stress or illness) and (2) do you drink fluids that have no sugar, measure your blood sugar again in 2 to 4 hours, check ketones if blood sugar is more than 300 mg/dl, and call the physician if your blood sugar is the same or higher or if ketones are moderate or large? Drawings such as the one in Figure 6-1 are meant to help patients remember symptoms of hypoglycemia and what the participant can do about them. Partipants

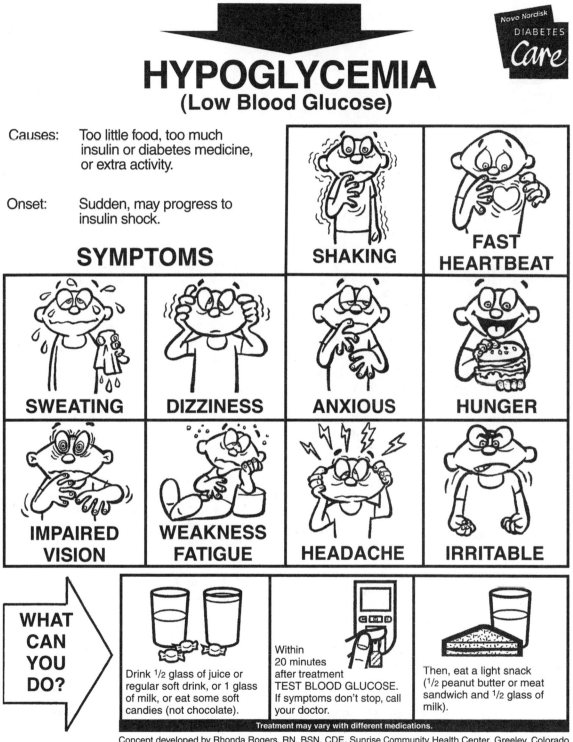

FIGURE **6-1** Detecting and managing hypoglycemia. From Novo Nordisk Pharmaceuticals, Inc., 2001, Greeley, Colorado.

practice reading food labels and following meal plans. Which of the following analogies used in this class do you think are helpful?

— Instructor explains insulin resistance by crossing her arms on her chest.
— High blood pressure damages blood vessels (instructor crushes plastic cup).
— Neuropathy is like when an animal chews the insulation (myelin) off an electrical cord (nerve).
— Amount of food is like a dose of medicine.

How are these stories helpful to others in the class?

— One partipant says she has had diabetes for 15 years and is now confused and distressed that what she was taught and followed religiously (no ice cream or sugar) is not what she's learning in this class.
— Another participant describes how she stepped on a tietack and didn't even feel it. She had a sore on her toe and in a day it was red and spreading to other toes. She had to have several toes amputated. Her message to other participants: do not underestimate how fast infections move.
— An instructor describes how a previous participant had a glycosylated hemoglobin (HbA$_{1c}$) of 14 when she came to the class, one of 8.7 three months after the class, and in 6 months it was 6.[1]

One participant doesn't say a word during the entire 9 hours of class and frequently has difficulty finding the right page in the workbook. What would you do?

GENERAL APPROACH

Diabetes education is the most fully developed of all the fields of patient education practice and among the oldest, having begun in the 1930s. Nationally accepted standards have been adopted for accrediting programs of diabetes education and for certification for an interdisciplinary advanced-practice role of certified diabetes educator (CDE) (see Appendix D). Because randomized clinical trials have shown that stringent blood glucose control is associated with decreased risk of complications,[1] intensive treatment is attempted to achieve glycemic control as close to the non-diabetic range as possible. Flexible adjustment

of insulin dose, frequent monitoring of glucose levels, diet and exercise instruction, and frequent counseling and dietary adjustments are important. The National Diabetes Education Program goals include (1) increasing public awareness of the seriousness of diabetes and its risk factors and prevention, (2) promoting effective self-management, (3) improving knowledge of diabetes among health professionals, and (4) promoting policies that improve quality of and access to diabetes care.[15]

Approximately 8% of all adults in the United States have diabetes, and the percentage is proportionally higher in Hispanic, American Indian, and African-American populations. Severe deficits in self-management skills such as glucose testing, diet, sick-day guidelines, and foot care have been identified in 50% to 80% of adults and children with diabetes. More than half of persons with diabetes receive limited or no diabetes self-management education.[2] In addition, significant shortfalls in the quality of care for diabetes leave a great deal of room for improvement.[11] For example, it is estimated that, although 20% to 25% of all hospitalized patients have diabetes, 40% of all people with diabetes who are hospitalized do not have diabetes listed on their hospital discharge record. Patients are often physiologically stressed during hospitalization (say for a coronary artery bypass graft) and as a result may require a more complex diabetes regimen after discharge. So, although persons with diabetes are dispersed throughout the hospital, they are not identified as having diabetes and frequently do not receive education during the hospitalization.[4]

EDUCATIONAL APPROACHES AND RESEARCH BASE

Several recent meta-analyses of studies on the effectiveness of diabetes education have been completed. All note that, because control groups receive considerable education, intervention effects are substantially underestimated. The measured outcome is usually HbA$_{1c}$, although many factors other than diabetes education affect it. Over a period of 10 years, every 1% decrease in this value decreases microvascular complications by 25% to 37%, the incidence of myocardial infarction by 14%, and the incidence of death related to diabetes by 21%.[17] Ellis and others[6] found the HbA_{1c} value on average to be .32 HbA_{1c} lower for groups receiving education, Gary and others,[8] and Hampson and others[10] among adolescents with type I diabetes and Norris and others.[17] Few of these studies demon-strated an effect of educational interventions on glycemic control longer than 3 to 6 months after baseline, leaving unanswered questions about longer-term impact.

Educational interventions can be described by (1) setting (1:1, group, patient, and family), (2) delivery (face-to-face, telecommunication, written literature), (3) teaching method (didactic, goal-setting dictated, goal-setting negotiated, situational problem solving, cognitive reframing), (4) content (diet, exercise, self-measurement of blood glucose, basic diabetes knowledge, medication adherence, psychosocial concerns), (5) degree to which the intervention is tailored to an initial assessment, and (6) intervention intensity (number and duration of episodes, intervention duration). In their summary of 31 studies, Norris and others[17] found that duration of contact between educator and patient was the only significant predictor of outcome; Ellis and others[6] found that dose or amount of intervention was not a sensitive indicator of its success or failure.

Modern diabetes self-management programs reflect a movement away from a goal of regimen compliance to a goal of patient empowerment. Such programs include a strong emphasis on self-efficacy and on the impact of diabetes on the totality of a person's life. Goals include enhancing the ability of patients to identify and set realistic goals, applying a systematic problem-solving process, managing the stress caused by living with diabetes, and identifying and obtaining appropriate social support. The view that patients should define their blood glucose targets, weighing the risk they are prepared to take and the efforts they are prepared to make, is heavily tempered by pressure to reduce complications.

Holmstrom and Rosenqvist's[12] study of Swedish patients shows how difficult it is for some to make the transition from compliance to self-management and empowerment. Some dutifully performed self-monitoring but did not understand what they were to do with the values; others believed monitored values occurred randomly. Yet the necessity of making this transition is apparent because of variability in how the disease is experienced and the necessity for daily and hourly management to meet the goal of euglycemia to control complications and improve daily life.

The data suggest that there are no symptoms consistently associated with hypoglycemia or hyperglycemia for all patients. Most patients appear to have one or more symptoms that are highly idiosyncratic, varying from patient to patient, and the patients are unaware of which symptoms are actually predictive in their own cases. A special form of training, called blood-glucose awareness training (BGAT), has been effective in teaching individuals with insulin-requiring diabetes to improve their ability to recognize blood glucose fluctuations. Patients use both internal cues (body feelings) and external cues (timing, type and amount of insulin, food, and exercise).

Blood glucose estimates made by adults in this way have been found to be accurate about 50% of the time but dangerously inaccurate 15% of the time, failing to detect hypoglycemia and hyperglycemia. BGAT involves teaching patients how to identify symptoms sensitive and specific to their hypoglycemia and hyperglycemia. At an average of 4.9 years after training, these patients had improved HbA_{1c} levels and had fewer automobile accidents than did control subjects who received routine diabetes education. Booster training (periodic brief retraining) was important. This work suggests that teaching classic signs or symptoms of hypoglycemia or hyperglycemia may be seriously misleading. Only one symptom (feeling shaky) was predictive of hypoglycemia for more than half of those studied, and in some cases a single symptom predicted hyperglycemia for one patient and hypoglycemia for another. Postintervention levels were still far from ideal.[3]

Depression is more prevalent in persons with diabetes than it is in the general population and it is associated with poor glycemic control and decreased compliance with therapy. Pharmacotherapy for depression may be poorly tolerated or insufficient to produce full remission in as many as half of persons with diabetes with major depression, or it may not be prescribed.[16] Depression makes learning and self-management difficult. Sixty percent of persons with diabetes report chronic pain, which also is significantly associated with poorer self-management[14] and difficulty in learning.

Teaching materials and approaches must reflect the fact that diabetes involves a complex regimen and often necessitates lifestyle changes on the part of a patient and family. Approaches must also be culturally sensitive. Brown's work in Starr County, Texas, was dscribed in Chapter 2. Other studies of a similar but low-income population found that patients commonly relied on medication as a safety valve to compensate for not following their diets. They ate "normal" foods until they had a crisis in glucose levels and then they ate more carefully until control was regained. Patients feared low rather than high blood glucose because of its distressing symptoms. Although patients knew what to do and were committed to taking care of themselves, many pushed the bounds of acceptable practice.[13]

Diabetes is a chronic and progressive disease. Particular transitions in self-management require special approaches; two examples are provided here. Because of progression in the underlying pathophysiologic mechanisms, the glycemic control through meal planning, physical activity, and oral medications that is effective in individuals newly diagnosed with type II diabetes generally cannot be maintained indefinitely. There is growing evidence that introducing basal insulin therapy earlier in the treatment course when oral agents are beginning to fail spares beta cell function. Introduction of insulin therapy often triggers a referral for diabetes education. Table 6-1 describes common concerns of these patients and strategies to address them.

Grey and others[9] describe training in coping skills, specifically tailored to help adolescents attain a sense of competence and mastery about social situations such as managing food choices with friends, decision making about drugs and alcohol, and independence/dependence conflicts. In groups of two to three individuals with a trainer, role playing is used to portray various social situations and modeling adaptive coping responses. After 3 months, youths receiving this training showed improved metabolic control and quality of life compared with those receiving intensive diabetes management alone sustained over a year.

Sarkadi and Rosenqvist's study[19] addressed three concerns that have been raised by research and practice, concerns that could have been expected in light of the issues about learning raised in Chapter 2. First, their program was entirely experience based and lasted long enough for participants to master necessary skills and judgments and to make them habits. The intervention was a 12-month group educational program based on participants' experience. During their monthly meetings, participants shared their self-monitoring diaries with the group and problems raised were solved by the group. Participants were encouraged to experiment with different nutritional components and exercise and to monitor their blood glucose reactions as a means to promote experienced-based learning. Second, participants were followed up for 24 months. At 1 year the experience-based group (in comparison with the wait-list control group) had a significant decrease in A1c levels, then a relapse, and at 2 years after baseline another decrease in HbA_{1c} levels (.4% decrease over baseline). This pattern shows that intervention effects may be postponed and may fluctuate. Third, patient satisfaction with their own diabetes knowledge was the best predictor of decreased HbA_{1c} 24 months after baseline.

A number of instruments are available to measure quality of life, attitudes, disease-relevant behaviors, and knowledge among children and adults with diabetes. These instruments may be found in the literature—ten are reproduced and critiqued in Redman.[18]

SUMMARY

Perhaps more than in any other area of practice, the success in patients with diabetes has demonstrated what can be accomplished with research, policies, standards, and services in support of self-management education. Yet large numbers of persons with this disorder are still not reached.

TABLE 6-1 Assessing and Addressing Common Concerns	
Common Concerns	**Strategies to Address Concerns**
Fear of needles or pain from injections	• Describe/show very fine needles • Offer insulin pens or other devices that hide the needle from view or may be less painful • Point out that injections are less painful than SMBG tests • Psychological counseling may be indicated
Fear of hypoglycemia	• Discuss insulin action times and minimal potential for hypoglycemia • Describe differences in risks for hypoglycemia between multiple and once-daily injections • Describe prevention strategies
Weight gain	• Educate about strategies to minimize weight gain (e.g., decreased caloric intake and increased exercise)
Adverse impact on lifestyle; inconvenient; loss of personal freedom and independence	• Discuss intensifying as a way to increase flexibility • Use once-daily insulin • Offer available resources and support
Belief that insulin means diabetes is worse or a more serious disease	• Review all treatment options as a progression from the beginning of education • Explain how insulin is a logical step in the progression as it relates to insulin resistance and beta cell failure
Insulin as personal failure	• Teach initially and review concept that beta cell failure is progressive • Avoid statements such as, "You've failed oral agents"; reframe statement as, "The oral agents have failed you." • Avoid using insulin as a threat to encourage weight loss and activity
Insulin causes complications	• Provide information about your experience with other people with diabetes • Present information about the UKPDS
Treated differently by family and friends	• Discuss support desired and how to ask for what is needed • Include family in education if requested by patient

SMBG, Self-monitoring of blood glucose levels; *UKPDS,* United Kingdom Prospective Diabetes Study.
(From Funnell MM, Kruger DF, Spencer M: Self-management support for insulin therapy in type 2 diabetes, *Diabetes Educ* 30:274-280, 2004.)

REFERENCES

1. Aubert RE and others: Nurse case management to improve glycemic control in diabetic patients in a health maintenance organization, *Ann Intern Med* 129:605-612, 1998.

2. Clement S: Diabetes self-management education, *Diabetes Care* 18:1204-1214, 1995.

3. Cox DJ and others: Long-term follow-up evaluation of blood glucose awareness training, *Diabetes Care* 17:1-5, 1994.

4. Davis ED: A quality improvement project in diabetes patient education during hospitalization. *Diabetes Spectrum* 13:228-231, 2000.

5. Detroit Medical Center: Outpatient diabetes education program, Detroit, MI.

6. Ellis SE and others: Diabetes patient education: a meta-analysis and meta-regression. *Patient Educ Couns* 42:97-105, 2004.

7. Funnell MM, Kruger DF, Spencer M: Self-management support for insulin therapy in type 2 diabetes, *Diabetes Educ* 30:274-280, 2004.

8. Gary TL, Genkiinger JM, Guallar E, Peyrot M, Brancati FL: Meta-analysis of randomized educational and behavioral interventions in type 2 diabetes. *Diabetes Educ* 29:488-501, 2003.

9. Grey M, Boland EA, Davidson M, Li J, Tamborlane WV: Coping skills training for youth with diabetes mellitus has long-lasting effects on metabolic control and quality of life, *J Pediatr* 137:107-113, 2000.

10. Hampson SE and others: Behavioral interventions for adolescents with type 1 diabetes, *Diabetes Care* 23:1416-1422, 2000.

11. Helseth LD, Susman JL, Crabtree PJ: Primary care physicians' perceptions of diabetes management, *J Fam Pract* 48:37-42, 1999.

12. Holmstrom IM, Rosenqvist U: Misunderstandings about illness and treatment among patients with type 2 diabetes, *J Adv Nurs* 49:146-154, 2005.

13. Hunt LM, Pugh J, Valenzuela M: How patients adapt diabetes self-care recommendations in everyday life, *J Fam Pract* 46:207-215, 1998.

14. Krein SL, Heisler M, Piette JD, Makki F, Kerr EA: The effect of chronic pain on diabetes patients' self-management, *Diabetes Care* 28:65-70, 2005.

15. Leontos C, Wong F, Gallivan J, Lising M: National Diabetes Education Program: Opportunities and challenges, *J Am Dietet Assoc* 98:73-75, 1998.

16. Lustman PJ and others: Cognitive behavior for depression in type 2 diabetes mellitus, *Ann Intern Med* 129:613-621, 1998.

17. Norris SL, Lau J, Smith SJ, Schmid CH, Engelgau MM: Self-management education for adults with type 2 diabetes, *Diabetes Care* 25:1159-1171, 2002.

18. Redman BK: *Measurement tools in patient education*, ed 2, New York, 2003, Springer.

19. Sarkadi A, Rosenqvist U: Experience-based group education in type 2 diabetes: a randomized controlled trial. *Patient Educ Couns* 53:291-298, 2004.

7

Education for Pregnancy and Parenting and Educating Children

CASE I

George[25] describes experiences of first-time mothers discharged from an acute-care hospital less than 48 hours after vaginal delivery. The mothers reported feeling well prepared for pregnancy, labor, and delivery but returned home feeling unprepared to care for themselves and their babies, overwhelmed, exhausted, unwell, and isolated. Many complained about the overwhelming amount of information offered in discharge teaching at the hospital and believed it concentrated primarily on care of the baby and not on care for themselves. Propelled into information seeking, they received conflicting and fragmented advice. Most felt uncomfortable initiating contact with a health professional about their concerns.

Is this outcome unusual? What learning/teaching conditions could explain these negative findings?

General Approach

Education for pregnancy, parenting, and educating children is an established field of practice in patient education.

Prenatal education is well incorporated into most maternity nursing texts and will not be revisited here. Prenatal care in the United States now routinely includes an offer of testing for chromosomal disorders and other genetic conditions; testing requires provision of adequate factual information as well as the support women and their partners need to make decisions that are both informed and autonomous. Prenatal testing decisions require simultaneous consideration of (1) the risk of giving birth to an affected child, (2) the risk of having an abnormal test result, and (3) the risk that the test may cause a pregnancy loss. Simple changes in the format used to present numerical risk information can influence perception and subsequent choices. Presentation of risk as the chance of having an affected child can result in a perception of higher risk and more testing than does presentation of risk as the chance of having an unaffected healthy child.[15]

Some educational efforts have focused on particular topics in detail. For example, the benefits of adequate levels of folic acid in decreasing the risk of neural tube defects were promoted by a mass media campaign particularly targeted at women of low socioeconomic status in the Netherlands. Although low-income women benefited from the campaign, those of higher income benefited more.[9] Special programs have been established to educate women who have positive test results for the hepatitis B virus during the prenatal period.[6]

The Resource Mothers program for women with maternal phenylketonuria (PKU) aims to increase positive outcomes for the babies by improving metabolic control. The majority of young women with PKU discontinue the restrictive diet during middle childhood and have difficulty resuming it, sometimes complicated by limited intellectual abilities and low socioeconomic status. In one population studied, more than 80% of pregnancies involved inadequate metabolic control. The Resource Mothers program includes 40 hours of instruction and home visitation to develop skills in cooking, shopping, meal planning, and preparation for the baby. The mean number of weeks it took to reach metabolic control was shorter in the studied intervention group than in the control group, and their babies were better developed.[32]

A special area of concern currently is patient education to aid in the early detection and treatment of preterm labor, which is part of a larger program of management. Of all preterm births, about 80% are the direct result of preterm labor, defined as the presence of uterine contractions with progressive cervical dilation or effacement, or both, occurring before 37 weeks' gestation. Programs for prevention have had inconsistent results in decreasing overall preterm birth rates, in part because risk-scoring systems still fall short of identifying most patients who have the problem. Goldenberg and Rouse[17] conclude that most medical interventions designed to prevent preterm birth, including patient education, do

not work. Despite this view, professional opinion still supports teaching patients to monitor for and promptly report symptoms of preterm labor (uterine contractions every 10 minutes or less, menstrual-like cramps, low dull backache, pelvic pressure, changes in vaginal discharge, urinary frequency, or intestinal cramping).[29] Women have found the symptoms ambiguous in that they were subtle, lacked a pattern, and unpredictably waxed and waned and thus were confused with the expected discomforts of pregnancy.

Postpartum learning needs documented over a number of studies showed that information about stitches, episiotomy, and postpartum complications were most important during the first three postpartum days, as was information about infant feeding and illness.[2] Education about postpartum fatigue and depression are also important.

Infant communication education, focusing on infant behaviors, states, and communication cues, has also been presented prenatally to first-time mothers, taught in part by videotape. This randomized controlled trial found significant differences in early mother-infant interaction, which is known to facilitate bonding and infant development.[26]

A special way of helping parents understand their baby's behavior is to demonstrate the Brazelton Neonatal Behavioral Assessment Scale (NBAS). This scale consists of 18 neurological reflexes and 28 behavioral items that examine the baby's interaction with his or her environment in four dimensions of functioning: autonomic stability, motor organization, state organization, and attention/interactive capacities. For example, reflexes (such as rooting and the Babinski reflex) and muscular assessments (such as pull-to-sit) test the infant's neuromuscular status. The baby possesses his or her own competencies, reportoire of coping skills, and individual responses to stressors and therefore has the capacity to influence reactions from caregivers in the environment. For example, the disorganized infant cannot restrain a response and may have an exaggerated reaction to gentle touch, thus responding with vigorous crying, which in turn may make caring for him or her difficult and place the baby at risk for neglect from caregivers who are intolerant or have poor coping skills. During the NBAS demonstration, parents are sensitized to their baby's uniqueness and develop a collaborative relationship with health care providers, using the baby's behavior as the language of communication.[14]

A meta-analysis of 13 studies of parenting interventions based on the NBAS showed an effect size of 0.4—a small to moderate beneficial effect—on quality of later parenting. The NBAS assesses an infant's alertness to auditory and visual stimuli, ability to tune out distraction, responses to stress, soothability, motor functioning, and reflexive behaviors.[21] It is administered by a trained examiner in the parent's presence, or the parents are trained to administer the instrument to their infants. In either case, the effect should be to educate the parent about the infant's capabilities.[7] Studies using the NBAS as a teaching tool have also shown strong results with groups such as depressed mothers.[21]

Attention to breast-feeding education remains high. Most women cease breast-feeding before the desired 6 to 12 months largely because they have difficulty with it. Consistent with learning theories outlined in Chapter 1, breast-feeding self-efficacy has been found to be predictive of those who continue to breast-feed and influenced by knowing others who have successfully done so (vicarious experience).[8] Trained peer counselors, operating under the supervision of a certified lactation consultant, were found in a low-income predominantly Latina population to yield higher breast-feeding rates than did routine breast-feeding education alone. The peer services included one prenatal visit, daily perinatal visits, three postpartum home visits, and telephone contact as needed, a considerable investment of time allowing practice, problem solving, and skill building.[4]

A meta-analysis of primary care–based interventions showed that education and support interventions to promote breast-feeding appear to improve its initiation and maintenance up to 6 months. Educational sessions that review the benefits of breast-feeding, principles of lactation, myths, common problems, solutions, and skills training appear to have the greatest single effect.

Common office and hospital practices of providing written materials and discharge packets have not been found to be effective in prompting breast-feeding.[19]

A developmentally oriented framework to understand what parents need to know flows from what is known about sensitive caregiving being critical in the development of a secure attachment relationship. Knowing the behavioral characteristics, strengths, and preferences of one's baby provides this foundation, as does understanding the infant state and its modulation and infant behaviors and cues. Infant state refers to the six levels of consciousness associated with coherent patterns of behavior. The full alert state is perfect for feeding, teaching, playing, and interacting. Over time, infants maintain this state for longer periods. Parents may benefit from a review of a range of interventions to arouse and soothe their infant as they learn what works best for their child. The pleasure and feeling of efficacy that comes from synchronous interaction with the infant is highly reinforcing to parents.[18]

Transition from the neonatal intensive care unit (NICU) to home is stressful for parents and requires concentrated instruction for them to become competent and confident in the care of the infant. Prematurity may have been the reason for NICU treatment; premature infants are often less responsive and more difficult to care for than are healthy term infants. Because of the immaturity of the central nervous system, these infants' behavior is more disorganized and unpredictable. They show less effective care-eliciting behavior and may not cry to signal the need for care, causing asynchrony in the parent-infant dyad, feeding is often characterized by slow food intake and excessive body movements or frequent spitting up, and they are more likely to have residual medical problems that require treatment at home.

Parents need to be taught basic caregiving, regulation of temperature, growth and development, and infant stimulation, and they must learn to recognize the signs and symptoms of illness, including abnormal breathing patterns. Despite agreement on discharge preparation needs, there is little evidence to indicate whether parents are currently being well prepared for

Box 7-1	*Positioning and Handling Techniques*

Positioning

- Horseshoe rolls (blankets made into a roll, shaped as a horseshoe, and placed around infant as boundaries)
- Head roll (blanket roll placed at top of bed so that, if infant pushes with legs, there is a boundary)
- Swaddling (with either blanket or T-shirt if infant is small)
- Sheepskin
- Hands to face

Handling

- Try to wake infant slowly (with soft touch or voice) before performing care.
- When performing caregiving activities, make sure infant remains in flexed position.
- Offer infant finger for grasping.
- Offer infant pacifier for nonnutritive sucking.
- If infant demonstrates various disengagement cues, give infant a break from the activity.

From Krebs TL: Clinical pathway for enhanced parent and preterm infant interaction through parent education, *J Perinat Neonatal Nurs* 12(2):38-49, 1998.

Box 7-2	*Infant Cues*

Disengagement Cues

- Hiccoughs
- Apnea
- Bradycardia
- Color changes
- Finger splaying
- Arching
- Extensions
- Grimacing

Engagement Cues

- Hands to midline
- Sucking
- Lip pucker
- Gazing
- Flexion
- Smiling
- Grasping

From Krebs TL: Clinical pathway for enhanced parent and preterm infant interaction through parent education, *J Perinat Neonatal Nurs* 12(2):38-49, 1998.

Box 7-3	*Environmental Enhancements*

Dim lights during day, provide dark environment at night
Use incubator cover to help modify lighting
Institute quiet time around bedside when infant is sleeping
Introduce music or parent tapes when infant is developmentally ready (≈33 to 35 weeks)
Place pictures of family at bedside for infant to look at when developmentally ready (≈33 to 35 weeks)
Cluster caregiving times

From Krebs TL: Clinical pathway for enhanced parent and preterm infant interaction through parent education, *J Perinat Neonatal Nurs* 12(2):38-49, 1998.

their infant's discharge. Boxes 7-1, 7-2, and 7-3 describe specific skills for positioning and handling, environmental enhancements, and reading of infant cues that these parents need to learn.[24] Interventions to facilitate parent-infant interactions include guiding parents to maximize periods of infant attentiveness and educating parents in specific interacting behaviors. Developmental delays are more likely in interaction mismatch—for example, when the parent continues to play despite the infant's overt behavioral signs of overstimulation. Outcome goals are for parents to (1) recognize their infants' engagement and disengagement cues, (2) respond appropriately to their infants' cues, and (3) perform caregiving activities according to their infants' cues.[25] Support groups for parents of preterm infants can help to normalize parental experiences and provide much needed information and family support.

Policies of most NICUs include teaching caretakers cardiopulmonary resuscitation (CPR) before discharge of the infant. These caretakers report decreased anxiety and increased feeling of control without an increased sense of responsibility and burden. It is important to remember that research has shown that within 6 months only one third of those educated at hospital discharge were able to perform CPR satisfactorily.[11,30] Thus periodic reassessment and reinstruction are important.

The Back to Sleep (BTS) campaign emphasizes placing healthy infants on their backs or sides to reduce the risk of sudden infant death syndrome (SIDS). The incidence of SIDS is two to three times higher in the African-American population compared with the U.S. population as a whole; prone sleeping is also twice as prevalent in African-American infants. Because BTS seems to have been less effective with this group, Moon and others[28] showed that a 15-minute educational intervention was effective in changing sleeping position practice among clients of the Women, Children, and Infants program. At 6 months after instruction, parents who attended were more likely to place their infants on their backs (75% vs 45%).

Traditional pediatric care is based on the assumption that parents have the basic knowledge and resources to provide a nurturing, safe environment. Free home visitation is a widespread early intervention strategy in most industrialized nations other than the United States. In England every prospective mother is visited at home at least once before birth with six more visits before the child is 5 years old. Special attention is focused on those in greater need of service, including mothers of low-birth-weight and premature children with chronic illness and disabilities, low-income unmarried teenage mothers, families with a history of substance abuse, and parents with a low intelligence quotient. The purpose of the visits is active promotion of positive health and infant caregiving and a decrease in family stress.[1] Parenting education programs for low-income parents of young children produce a significant decrease in verbal and corporal punishment and a significant increase in nurturing behaviors, with children's behavior improving significantly. The abusive parent has been characterized as having low tolerance for frustration, impaired parenting skills, a sense of incompetence in parenting, unrealistic expectations of children, inappropriate expression of anger, and social isolation.[13]

A long-term follow-up of nurse home visitation (seven home visits during pregnancy and 26 from birth to child's second birthday) showed that, compared with a control group, those visited had fewer subsequent pregnancies, longer intervals between birth of first and second children, and fewer months using public assistance. The nurses followed detailed visit-by-visit guidelines to help women improve their health-related behaviors, care of their children, and life course development such as pregnancy planning, educational achievement, and workforce participation. The women set small, achievable behavioral objectives that, when met, increased their confidence in their ability to manage greater challenges.[24]

National Standards and Testing Programs

Both childbirth educators and lactation consultants can be certified through international associations. Other certifications are also available.

CASE II

Rose is a 4-year-old girl admitted to the preoperative area of a children's hospital to have her adenoids removed. She clings to her mother, hiding her face, and is unwilling to allow the nurse to measure her vital signs or to acknowledge the child life specialist (CLS) who is present to prepare her for surgery. The CLS rubs Rose's hand and eventually gets her to watch a video of the character Dora. Twenty minutes later the child is on the floor fashioning a heart with a modeling clay cutter. Eventually, before Rose goes to surgery, the CLS gets her to medical play, which will directly prepare her for her surgery experience. She phones the physician and suggests that this patient is highly anxious and would benefit from preoperative midazolam. The CLS uses the following principles in her work: always give the child choices, use play to normalize the experience, and help the child cope.

CASE III

Eleven-year-old Angela is in hospital for revision of her hydrocephalus shunt, having come in through the emergency department. Although the family wanted the shunt removed, they were persuaded that

Angela still needed it. There are four younger children in the family. Dad cannot read. The nurse specialist is preparing the patient and family for discharge and hands the mom the book *About Hydrocephalus: A Book for Families* published by the Hydrocephalus Association. The nurse rattles off how long the shunt is to allow the child to grow, symptoms to watch for if the shunt goes bad, not to allow the child to go on a roller coaster, and not to allow the child to bathe for a specified period of time. The mom nods her head to all of this. Dad asks if the child can go on vacation. Do you have any idea whether this family knows what to do? They've successfully cared for Angela's shunt since it was first put in and seem confident in their ability to do so now.

EDUCATING CHILDREN

General Approach

Theory and research about how children learn are presented in Chapter 2. In addition, several earlier chapters include examples of education for health problems, such as asthma, that commonly affect children. Some earlier sections of this chapter that focus on education for parenting also include an educational component for children. This section provides examples of how patient education services primarily focused on children are being offered in communities and health care institutions with a particular focus on asthma.

Educational Approaches and Research Base

Consider children with myelomeningoceles, who must learn self-catheterization because of a neurogenic bladder. The goal is to promote continence and prevent renal deterioration and to significantly decrease the incidence of bacteriuria. Girls have to be able to perform the psychomotor skills of washing hands, gathering equipment, removing garments, washing the perineum, lubricating the catheter, spreading the labia and inserting the catheter, draining the bladder, removing the catheter, and washing the catheter and hands. Teaching involves an anatomically correct doll placed in the child's lap face forward,

guiding the child to become proficient in use of the catheter with the doll and then with herself. Appropriate reinforcement is important.[33]

Or consider preparing 4- to 8-year-old children for a magnetic resonance imaging (MRI) procedure with its narrow bore tube and noise for a period of time. Because sedation and anesthesia can be as frightening as the procedure, an alternate play therapy preparation was developed. Teaching involved explaining the procedure in age-appropriate terms. Photos of children or a teddy bear undergoing MRI emphasize what the examination entails and what the child is required to do. A small model of an MRI unit including sliding table top and light and a tape recording of the noise allows children to act out the examination and play with plastic figures representing themselves, the radiographers, and nurses. A color-in storybook of a visit to the MRI unit through the eyes of a child is used. Although apparently no control group was studied, the authors believe there has been a dramatic decrease in the number of failed MRI examinations.[31]

Asthma provides a good example of a disease that heavily affects children (four million to 14 years of age), can be life threatening, is chronic, and must be self-managed by family and children over a long period of time through many developmental changes. This disease disproportionately affects minority and poor children, with higher levels of morbidity and mortality. The National Asthma Education and Prevention Program (NAEP) released practice guidelines in 1997 based on current research and expert consensus. A study of children with asthma in two managed care organizations found deficiencies in meeting NAEP guidelines in many areas of care but particularly in patient education in how to adjust medications before exposures, written instructions for management of asthma attacks, and regular use of long-term control medication.[10] Asthma education programs have reduced emergency department visits and hospitalizations, decreased school absences, and improved school performance.[3]

Particular instructional problem areas are well known. Many asthmatic children use their inhaler devices too poorly to result in reliable drug delivery, even after inhalation instruction. Comprehensive inhalation instruction until the trainer is satisfied and repeated checkups are needed. The common approach of a single short instruction session on the use of an inhaler device is unlikely to be successful.[23] Explanatory models for asthma among school-age children frequently focus on contagion. Half of the mothers of these children thought all their child's medications had similar functions, discontinued some because they thought their child was being given too much medication, and thought the asthma would go away. These beliefs and explanatory models must be elicited and addressed because they direct care actions.[20]

Teaching abstract concepts such as inflammation to children is difficult because their thinking is characterized by concrete operations. Meng and McConnell[27] describe a 3-foot-tall, lifelike doll whose chest opens to reveal ribs, which can be removed to reveal the surface of the lungs, trachea, and main bronchi. The right lung opens to reveal healthy bronchi, bronchioles, and air sacs. The left chest contains inflamed lungs that open to expose red airways that bulge around smooth muscles. A pocket contains a miniature bronchiole that, when inflated, swells, causing occlusion of the airway. Yellow-green synthetic mucus is added to the inside of the tube. A balloon can be used to simulate a wheeze. Children are asked to identify the symptoms they experience when their asthma flares up. Use of rescue and controller medications is linked to smooth muscles and an open airway. The teacher explains that the doll (Randy) has learned to take his controller medication every day and now revisits his friend with the cat.

Community sites for delivery of asthma education to children help to make it available and incorporated into their everyday lives. Brown and others[3] describe a home visiting asthma education program for children less than 7 years old. The Wee Wheezers at Home program consists of eight 90-minute educational sessions to be delivered at weekly intervals to low-income families. Families receive printed materials tailored to a fifth grade reading level and are assigned homework at each lesson.

Much more common are programs delivered through the school system. A historical review of these programs may be found in Christiansen and Zuraw.[5] One such program is the Open Airways for Schools (OAS) program, which has been shown to improve the self-management skills and health outcomes of students with asthma in grades 3 to 5. More recent work shows that children's participation in OAS was a significant predictor of parental self-management skills, which means that children can teach their parents about asthma. Parents did not directly take part in the six 60-minute sessions in which groups of eight to 12 children learned new asthma self-management skills. Practice and feedback in class, reinforcement for use of the skills, use of stories and artistic activities, and role play to rehearse asthma management skills were used; a variety of instructional techniques were also used. The program involved parents by assigning homework for the child to carry out with parents and siblings. Learning objectives of the program are to teach children to (1) recognize the onset of asthma symptoms, (2) begin self-management steps immediately, and (3) recognize the signs that emergency care is needed. In comparison with controls, children who took part in the program had improved self-management skills, self-efficacy, school performance, and quality of life and asthma symptoms significantly less often.[12]

Another great example is a school-based asthma disease management program of National Jewish Hospital in Denver, Colorado. Children receive monthly asthma education at school with access to an online program. Each child participating in the program received two peak flowmeters—one for school and one for home—and training in their use. The child recorded peak flow readings, symptoms, asthma-related activity such as physician and emergency department visits and rescue medication usage daily into a confidential, computerized interactive Internet diary on the school's computer, assisted by a respiratory nurse or therapist. Alerts would come from care managers at National Jewish who monitored the diaries on a daily basis. Children could send e-mail directly to the Asthma Wizard at National Jewish. Parents received several educational calls about asthma and had a 24/7 emergency number to call if problems arose. At 6 months, missed school days and unscheduled physician visits were decreased by two thirds, daytime symptoms by 62% and nighttime symptoms by 34%.[34]

SUMMARY

Pregnancy, parenting, and child development offer many opportunities for teaching that will make a real difference in people's lives, yet little evidence is found to indicate whether these opportunities are exploited. Much work remains to be accomplished in the development of standards of practice and tested programs.

Study Questions

1. Because children who have been critically ill may be at increased risk for a respiratory or cardiac event at home, it is important that the parents learn basic life-support skills. What learning conditions are essential so that the parents are competent and feel confident in providing this care for their child?
2. In the box to the right, a nurse describes her work with a premature baby and his mother. Identify the learning principles involved.
3. The BTS campaign has disseminated the message that infants should sleep in a supine position. Studies found decreases in the prone sleep positioning from 70% in 1992 to 24% in 1996 and in rates of SIDS from 1.2 to 0.74 per 1000 live births. A more recent telephone survey of African-American, Hispanic, Asian, and American Indian parents from inner cities in the north central United States found that, although 80% of these parents had heard of sleep position recommendations, 40% still preferred prone positioning. Parents feared that choking would occur in the supine position and felt their infants slept better on their stomachs. The authors indicated that more efforts are needed to convince parents who disagree with and resist recommendations.[22] How would you do this?

"One of our mothers was frightened and unsure about holding her baby. Stating that she didn't know how and was afraid that he would choke, the mother would try to feed her son, but then quickly hand him over to the nurse. As the developmental specialist, I sat down with the mother and refused to let her hand her son over. Instead, I encouraged her to watch his mouth, counting his breaths and watching his sucking and swallowing. I suddenly noticed that her baby had stopped sucking and was staring at her face, scanning the outer edges of her head in an arch. I whispered to her to look at her baby's face. When she saw the intense focus and clear interest in his face, she melted and was enthralled. As she smiled, her baby continued to look at her. I suggested that she remain still so that he could scan her face. From that moment on, her behavior changed. She began to watch him closely and then asked him if he was ready to eat. When she saw the clear, alert look, she knew he was ready. She even learned that if she shifted her face away, he could suck more easily and that if she brought it back during his breaks, he rested and relaxed while gazing at her. No longer was she afraid."

Learning Principles

_____
_____
_____
_____
_____
_____
_____
_____
_____

From VandenBerg KA: What to tell parents about the developmental needs of their baby at discharge, *Neonatal Network* 18:57-59, 1999.

REFERENCES

1. American Academy of Pediatrics: The role of home-visitation programs in improving health outcomes in children and families, *Pediatrics* 101:486-489, 1998.
2. Bowman KG: Postpartum learning needs, *JOGNN* 34:438-443, 2005.

3. Brown JV and others: A home visiting asthma education program: Challenges to program implementation, *Health Educ Behav* 32:42-56, 2005.

4. Chapman DJ, Damio G, Young S, Perez-Wscamilla R: Effectiveness of breastfeeding peer counseling in a low-income, predominantly Latina population, *Arch Pediatr Adolesc Med* 158:897-902, 2004.

5. Christiansen SC, Zuraw BL: Serving the underserved: School-based asthma intervention programs, *J Asthma* 39:463-472, 2002.

6. Corrarino JE, Walsh PJ, Anselmo D: A program to educate women who test positive for the hepatitis B virus during the perinatal period, *Am J Matern Child Nurs* 24:151-155, 1999.

7. DasEilen R, Reifman A: Effects of Brazelton demonstrations on later parenting: a meta-analysis, *J Pediatr Psychol* 21:857-868, 1996.

8. Dennis CL: Theoretical underpinnings of breastfeeding confidence: A self-efficacy framework, *J Ilum Lact* 15:195-201, 1999.

9. DeWalle HEK and others: Effect of mass media campaign to reduce socioeconomic differences in women's awareness and behavior concerning use of folic acid: Cross sectional study, *BMJ* 319:291-292, 1999.

10. Diette GB and others: Consistency of care with national guidelines for children with asthma in managed care, *J Pediatr* 138:59-64, 2001.

11. Dracup K, Doering LV, Moser DK, Evangelista L: Retention and use of cardiopulmonary resuscitation skills in parents of infants at risk for cardiopulmonary arrest, *Pediatr Nurs* 24:219-225, 1998.

12. Evans D, Clark NM, Levinson MJ, Levin B, Mellins RB: Can children teach their parents about asthma? *Health Educ Behav* 28:500-511, 2001.

13. Fennell DC, Fishel AH: Parent education: an evaluation of STEP on abusive parents' perceptions and abuse potential, *J Child Adolesc Psychiatr Nurs* 11:107-120, 1998.

14. Fowles ER: The Brazelton Neonatal Behavioral Assessment Scale and maternal identity, *MCN Am J Matern Child Nurs* 24:287-293, 1999.

15. Gates EA: Communicating risk in prenatal genetic testing, *J Midwifery Womens Health* 49:220-227, 2004.

16. George L: Lack of preparedness: Experiences of first-time mothers, *MCN Am J Matern Child Nurs* 30:251-255, 2005.

17. Goldenberg RL, Rouse DJ: Prevention of premature birth, *N Engl J Med* 339:313-320, 1998.

18. Gottesman MM: Enabling parents to "read" their baby, *J Pediatr HealthCare* 13:148-151, 1999.

19. Guise J and others: The effectiveness of primary care–based interventions to promote breastfeeding: Systematic evidence review and meta-analysis for the US Preventive Services Task Force, *Ann Fam Med* 1:70-78, 2003.

20. Handelman L, Rich M, Bridgemohan CF, Schneider L: Understanding pediatric inner-city asthma: An explanatory model approach, *J Asthma* 41:166-177, 2004.

21. Hart S, Field T, Nearing G: Depressed mothers' neonates improve following the MABI and a Brazelton demonstration, *J Pediatr Psychol* 23:351-356, 1998.

22. Johnson CM and others: Infant sleep position: a telephone survey of inner-city parents of color, *Pediatrics* 104:1208-1211, 1999.

23. Kamps AWA, vanEwijk B, Roorda RJ, Brand PLP: Poor inhalation technique, even after inhalation instructions, in children with asthma, *Pediatr Pulmonol* 29:39-42, 2000.

24. Kitzman H and others: Enduring effects of nurse home visitation on maternal life course, *JAMA* 283:1983-1989, 2000.

25. Krebs TL: Clinical pathway for enhanced parent and preterm infant interaction through parent education, *J Perinat Neonat Nurs* 12:38-49, 1998.

26. Leitch DB: Mother-infant interaction: Achieving synchrony, *Nurs Res* 48:55-58, 1999.

27. Meng A, McConnell S: Asthma education: special applications for the school-age child, *Nurs Clin North Am* 38:653-664, 2003.

28. Moon RY, Oden RP, Grady KC: Back to sleep: An educational intervention with women, infants and children program clients, *Pediatrics* 113:542-547, 2004.

29. Moore ML, Freda MC: Reducing preterm and low birth-weight births: Still a nursing challenge, *Matern Child Nurs* 23:200-208, 1998.

30. Moser DK, Dracup K, Doering LV: Effect of cardiopulmonary resuscitation training for parents of high-risk neonates on perceived anxiety, control and burden, *Heart Lung* 28:326-333, 1999.

31. Pressdee D, May L, Eastman E, Grier D: The use of play therapy in the preparation of children undergoing MR imaging, *Clin Radiol* 52:945-947, 1997.

32. St. James PS, Shapiro E, Waisbren SE: The resource mothers program for maternal phenylketonuria, *Am J Public Health* 89:762-764, 1999.

33. Segal ES, Deatrich JA, Hagelgans NA: The determinants of self-catheterization programs in children with myelomeningoceles, *J Pediatr Nurs* 10:82-88, 1995.

34. Tinkelman D, Schwartz A: School-based asthma disease management, *J Asthma* 41:455-462, 2004.

8

Other Areas of Patient Education Practice

This chapter describes several fields of patient education practice that are in various stages of development.

RHEUMATIC DISEASES

Osteoarthritis affects 50% to 80% of the elderly population and rheumatoid arthritis (RA) 1% to 3% of the adult population; clearly these disorders are a source of significant pain and disability.

The Arthritis Self-Management Program (ASMP) has been constantly improved since its initial development in 1978, using lay leaders and an interactive, participatory style. Course content includes (1) knowledge about the major types of arthritis, nutrition, and use of medication; (2) skills for improving function, decreasing pain and negative emotions through the use of cognitive restructuring techniques and physical activity; (3) problem solving for health-related problems; and (4) techniques for improving communication with family and physicians. Randomized trials have shown that ASMP increases self-efficacy, self-management (SM) behaviors, exercise, and

use of cognitive management techniques to decrease pain, and it decreases ambulatory visits to physicians. Longitudinal cohort studies have demonstrated that these effects continue without formal reinforcement for as long as 4 years.[16]

A recent study compared a mail-delivered tailored SM intervention (SMART) with the classic ASMP and found both to be effective. Compared with usual-care patients, SMART participants had significantly decreased disability, improved role function, and increased self-efficacy at 1 year follow-up and decreases in global severity and physician visits and increases in self-efficacy at 2-year follow-up. SMART is tailored specifically to the exact diagnosis, problems, symptoms, demographics, health status, medications, self-efficacy, and other personal features of the patient. Because no reimbursement has been available for SM programs and previous models were labor intensive, large numbers of patients could not access them. The ASMP is readily replicated although it requires a local management structure and trained leaders. SMART can be delivered broadly from a centralized location at any time but requires extensive computer support at a cost of $100 per patient per year.[15]

The Spanish Arthritis Empowerment Program, a culturally adapted ASMP, has been tested in southern and northern California in largely immigrant populations with 55% having a sixth grade education or less and 60% having no medical insurance. Significant improvement in pain, self-efficacy, self-care behavior, arthritis knowledge, and general health was documented from pretest to 6-month follow-up.[26]

There is evidence that studies using only patients with RA show a smaller effect than studies with patients with other rheumatic diseases or with mixed study populations. Patients with recent-onset disease have been shown to benefit the most from patient education; in the long term there was no improvement in health status.[19] A Cochrane review of 50 studies found modest statistically significant benefits of patient education on functional disability at first follow-up, enabling patients to perform tasks more easily and with less pain. By final follow-up (3-14 months) there were no significant benefits. Outcomes such as fatigue and social participation may better capture benefits of patient education.[22]

Study of a joint protection SM program for persons with RA that used skills practice, goal setting, and home assignments showed significant improvement in joint protection and functional ability. Deformities did not develop as frequently in the joint protection group. This approach teaches patients how to alter methods and movement patterns of affected joints by use of assistive devices and pacing activities to reduce pain, inflammation, and stresses applied to joints during daily activity.[9]

A review of 17 studies that included patient education for both osteoarthritis and RA but focused on pain and disability found small reductions in both.[24]

MENTAL HEALTH

The mental health field has developed what it calls "psychoeducation," which refers to training individuals in psychological knowledge and skills, similar to what is called "patient education" in other fields. Originally used with persons with schizophrenia, this model is now applied to individuals with depression and bipolar disorder, to those with serious mental illness, and to those with obsessive-compulsive disorder.

Psychoeducation provides knowledge and skill development and support for individuals with mental illness and for their families. The family is especially important because the environment it creates (high expressed emotion, negative affective style) can influence the course of illness and recovery for the patient and because family members themselves need help in coping with the negative effects of the illness. The purposes of patient and family psychoeducation include ameliorating symptoms of the illness; reducing family burden and stress; helping participants acquire new coping, social, and communication skills that will improve their quality of life; enhancing treatment compliance; and relapse prevention and warning.

More than thirty randomized controlled trials (RCT) have demonstrated decreased relapse rates, improved recovery of patients, and family well-being from family psychoeducation. Common elements in these programs include education, including development of problem-solving skills and communication skills, continuing support, and clinical resources during periods of crisis. Again, information alone fails to decrease relapse rates. The focus is on educating and persuading families that how they behave toward the patient can facilitate or impede recovery. Meeting needs of family members also dramatically improves patient outcomes. Although family psychoeducation has a deep enough research base to be considered an evidence-based practice, it is rarely offered.[17] The group leader for a psychoeducational group needs to be able to tolerate the slow pace and frequent repetitions of content as well as patients' internal states of depression. An example of educational sessions for a psychoeducational intervention for persons with bipolar disorder may be seen in Box 8-1.[21]

Prevention of relapse is a prime educational goal for persons with bipolar disorder or with schizophrenia. Perry and others[20] taught patients with bipolar disorder (manic-depressive disorder)

Box 8-1	*Sessions of the Psycho-educational Intervention*

Understanding the nature of the illness
Manic and hypomanic episodes: Main symptoms and early identification of procedures
Depressive and mixed episodes: Main symptoms and early identification of prodromes
Identification of triggering factors
Treatment: Mood stabilizers
Family and treatment: Antipsychotics and antidepressants
Family and treatment: Enhancing compliance
Planning of coping strategies
Other important issues: Suicidal thoughts, hospitilization, rapid cycling, pregnancy, and counseling on genetic factors
Prevention and management of family stress: Communication skills
Prevention and management of family stress: Problem solving
Legal and social resources

Reinares M and others: Impact of a psychoeducational family intervention on caregivers of stabilized bipolar patients, *Psychother Psychosom* 73:312-319, 2004, with permission of S. Karger AG, Basel.

to identify early symptoms of relapse, which are frequently idiosyncratic to the patient and usually occur 2 to 4 weeks before full relapse. This approach did not work with depressive cycles but did significantly extend time between manic relapses in comparison with a control group. Persons with schizophrenia learn the relationship between illness and stress, including its link to relapse; medication taking; legal issues including patient rights; identification of early symptoms of acute episodes; and communication, problem solving and negotiation skills.[14]

Persons with chronic mental illness have a higher prevalence of medical illnesses and higher mortality rates than in the general population. They are expected to manage their own medical care although the symptoms of their disorders—hallucinations, delusions, paranoia, and withdrawal

from depression—may interfere with their ability to seek health care and to follow through with recommendations. Frequently, lack of knowledge, home, family, or network of friends are barriers to self-care for general health problems.[5]

A report of an 8-week patient education program for posttraumatic stress disorder appears to be a first. Posttraumatic stress disorder is an anxiety disorder that can ensue after exposure to life-threatening accidents, injuries that elicit intense fear, helplessness, or horror followed by persistent re-experiencing of the event. It has been shown to be associated with significant medical and psychiatric comorbidity. Treatment requires patients to eliminate coping strategies such as avoidance behaviors, which are comforting in the short-run but serve to maintain the disorder, in favor of behaviors that are transiently distressing but necessary for long-term decrements in anxiety. This requires that patients fully understand the etiology of the disorder, the corresponding rationale for treatment, reasonable expectations (complete symptom relief is atypical), and use of alcohol and illicit substances as a coping mechanism. Gray and others[8] developed this pilot patient education program for a group of combat veterans.

PREPROCEDURE AND POSTPROCEDURE EDUCATION

CASE

You observe Carol teach a total knee surgery preoperative class. She also makes rounds of the patients when they are in for surgery and then does home follow-up, providing reinforcement of a consistent set of messages, philosophy about learning, and comforting support. Personal Recovery Coaches (family members) attend class with patients. Ninety percent of the patients undergoing this surgery at this hospital attend Carol's class. Although the expense for the class is about $80, for which the hospital is not reimbursed, the class is free. Carol teaches with Power Point slides, using photos of actual providers in the units. She focuses on helping patients understand what they want from the surgery, coaching them to form realistic outcomes.

The class is focused on what patients will experience. Carol uses her knee to show bandages, drain and ice compression therapy, demonstrates walking stairs, getting on and off the toilet, and leg exercises. She explains the potential for developing a blood clot in the leg and shows patients how to give themselves the injection meant to prevent the clot. Exercises; positioning; and bed, tub, and car transfers are demonstrated and diagrams are available in teaching materials given to all patients.

This is the best class I have ever observed!!

Two RCTs of patient education for hip surgery support investment of the hospital in the case above, for providing the class. The first found that patients receiving education were significantly less anxious before surgery, had less pain, and were able to stand sooner than those who did not receive education.[6] The second study combined education with rehabilitation and found a reduction in hospital stay by 3 days, higher levels of satisfaction, and more realistic expectations of surgery among the experimental group.[18] Yet another investigator used a Web site to provide preoperative information, enhanced with digital photos and bookmarked so patients could log on easily. Patients in the experimental group used the Web site in addition to formal patient education and showed a significant increase in learning test scores.[11]

Preprocedure and postprocedure education encompasses a wide variety of medical treatments, including surgery. A relatively strong research base has developed around the use of sensory information (what the patient will see, hear, feel, smell, and taste) during the procedure and procedural information (description of what will be done during the procedure) to help patients minimize their emotional reactions, increase their coping strategies, and have a better outcome from the procedure. The optimal amount of each kind of information has not been established. Self-regulation theory, a cognitive theory that explains human behavior as an outcome of information processing, is the basis for research on preparatory teaching. A schema (mental image based on prior experience) serves as a framework for organizing input as an experience progresses, and teaching sensory and procedural information helps to develop the schema about the event.

An RCT found that patients who received a preoperative video were two to 16 times more likely to be able to recall appropriate knowledge than were those receiving usual care. The video relieves caregivers of step-by-step explanations of the procedure and allows them to focus on individual concerns and needs of a patient.[3] In another RCT Bondy and others[1] found that mailing a video and pamphlets to the patient's home to provide anesthetic-focused patient education for total hip and total knee replacement surgery diminished the preoperative anxiety in comparison with the normal procedure of using a clinical pathway and a visit with an anesthetist. The video showed the sequence of events before, during, and after anesthesia and explained benefits and possible side effects. Such an outcome is important because it can decrease the need for sedation to relieve anxiety and pain.[1]

Patient-controlled analgesia (PCA) is most frequently initiated in the recovery room when patients are emerging from general anesthesia; it may not have been planned preoperatively. Inclusion of PCA education in all preoperative education would solve this problem. Those who have been formally educated had lower pain intensity scores.[12] Because there is a temporary decrease in cognitive ability in the immediate postoperative period, which is to be expected because some of the drugs used were developed especially to produce amnesia of the intraoperative episode, it is important to teach PCA preoperatively. Studies have shown that PCA can yield higher levels of patient satisfaction with less sedation, shorter lengths of stay, and fewer complications.[25]

As ambulatory surgery has become increasingly common and hospital stays shorter, the burden of responsibility for preoperative and postoperative management has shifted to patient and family. For safe care, they must be well educated.

WOMEN'S HEALTH PATIENT EDUCATION

For some conditions in women's health education (primarily those affecting older women) educational programs have been found helpful.

Osteoporosis affects 13% to 18% of postmenopausal white women in the United States and lesser percentages of nonwhite women and men. The combination of medication, good nutrition including calcium and vitamin D, weight-bearing and muscle-strengthening exercise, and calcium supplements can reduce the rate of bone loss and promote the development of normal bone tissue. Davis and White[2] describe a 4-week osteoporosis education program for older adults in a residential setting. Teaching approaches included knowing calcium content of selected foods, completing individual assignments of dietary intake assessment and goal setting, having an opportunity to discuss progress individuals were making toward their goals, and reinforcing previous content using game questions on a large posterboard with answers underneath.

Osteoporosis education can be delivered in many settings. An RCT using a 10-minute video about ways to prevent bone loss shown before office visits found significantly more of those receiving this intervention start to take calcium supplements and hormone therapy in comparison with a control group that saw the physician in a routine manner.[13] It is important to note that many women have now chosen not to use hormone replacement therapy for this purpose because of side effects. An RCT of education and questions to ask their physicians, provided to women with hip fractures during hospitalization, found that those who received it were more likely to receive appropriate therapy than was the control group. Despite the known relationship between osteoporosis and hip fractures, patients who sustain one are grossly underdiagnosed and undertreated for osteoporosis.[4]

Another topic of importance to women's health is urinary incontinence, which affects 30% to 50% of community-dwelling older women. Behavioral therapy is most commonly used, including assisted toileting, bladder training, and pelvic muscle rehabilitation including pelvic muscle exercises. These modalities are hypothesized to improve bladder control by teaching patients how to control the physiologic responses of the bladder and pelvic muscles that mediate continence. One fourth to one half of women achieve near continence with behavior therapy,

which is similar to the efficacy of pharmacologic therapy. An RCT of six weekly instructional sessions on bladder training with individualized voiding schedules showed a 50% reduction in the mean number of incontinent episodes compared with a 15% reduction for control subjects who received no instruction but kept urinary diaries. Incontinence is often diagnosed by primary care providers who could immediately begin low-intensity behavioral therapy.[23]

New information is also available for self-management for women with irritable bowel syndrome, which affects 10% to 17% of women in industrialized nations. A three-arm RCT including a comprehensive eight-session intervention including education and reassurance, diet, relaxation and cognitive behavioral therapy; a condensed version of one 90-minute session; and a control group of usual care was performed by Heitkemper and others.[10] The comprehensive intervention included homework assignments and, beginning with those that allowed participants to succeed, reinforcement, and rehearsal of assignments; the intervention taught women which signs and symptoms were important to consult a health professional, how to recognize foods associated with their symptoms, assertiveness and social skills training, and cognitive restructuring including writing down automatic thoughts and using alternate ones. Cognitive behavior therapy is based on the hypothesis that irritable bowel syndrome symptoms are due, at least in part, to inappropriate cognitions about visceral sensations. Compared with usual care, women in the comprehensive program had reduced gastrointestinal symptoms, psychological distress, and interruption in activities because of symptoms and enhanced quality of life; the brief intervention did not improve symptoms. It is important to note that patient education was one of several psychosocial therapies used and that practice, skills training, and presumably development of confidence in controlling symptoms were important.

SUMMARY

This chapter describes areas of patient eduction practice that range from those that are just developing to those

---

| **Box 8-2** | *Goals for Teaching Home Mechanical Ventilation Care* |

1. Maintain Clear Airway

Education related to:
Tracheostomy care, suctioning, tube change
Signs of infection
Proper hydration for thin, clear secretions
Chest physiotherapy and augmented cough
Medication administration: Bronchodilators
　and antibiotics
Mobility

**2. Maintain Adequate Oxygenation and
Ventilation**

Education related to:
Proper use and maintenance of mechanical
　ventilator
Use of manual resuscitation bag
In-line nebulized medications

**3. Perform Skills to Maintain Cleanliness and
Maximum Strength and Flexibility**

Education related to:
Bathing, shampooing, shaving
Mouth care
Management of bowel and bladder elimination
Range-of-motion, strength, and flexibility
　exercises

**4. Prevent Irritation, Infection, and Skin
Breakdown**

Education related to:
Turning, positioning
Transfer, ambulation
Tracheostomy stoma care, PEG site care

5. Maintain Adequate Nutrition and Hydration

Education related to:
Feeding
Flushing, declogging tube
Assessing hydration/dehydration
Recognizing and dealing with diarrhea and
　constipation

**6. Maintain Effective Coping with Home Care for
Both Patient and Caregivers**

Education related to:
Recognition of coping skills found to be useful
　in past experiences
Communication
Resources for counseling, networking with
　others
Other care options available

From Glass C, Grap MJ, Battle G: Preparing the patient and family for home mechanical ventilation, *Med Surg Nurs*
8:99-107, 1999.
PEG, Percutaneous endoscopic gastrostomy.

---

with a stable research base, the findings of which should be widely applied in practice.

Study question

1. Home mechanical ventilation has emerged as a method for treating chronic stable respiratory failure, particularly from neuromuscular disease. Families spend an average of 11 hours a day providing care, which includes maintaining adequate caloric intake and a workable bowel program, responding to alarms, and developing skills for cleaning the ventilator, performing manual resuscitation in case of equipment shutdown, preventing aspiration,

etc. Box 8-2 describes goals for teaching home mechanical ventilation care.[17] Critique this plan.

REFERENCES

1. Bondy LR and others: The effect of patient education on preoperative patient anxiety, *Regl Anesth Pain Med* 24:158-164, 1999.
2. Davis GC, White TL: Planning an osteoporosis education program for older adults in a residential setting, *J Gerontol Nurs* 26:16-23, 2000.
3. Done ML, Lee A: The use of a video to convey preanesthetic information to patients undergoing ambulatory surgery, *Anesth Analg* 87:531-536, 1998.
4. Gardner MJ and others: Interventions to improve osteoporosis treatment following hip fracture: A prospective randomized trial, *J Bone Joint Surg* 87:3-7, 2005.

5. Getty C, Perese E, Knaub S: Capacity for self-care of persons with mental illnesses living in community residences and the ability of their surrogate families to perform health care functions, *Issues Ment Health Nurs* 19:53-70, 1998.

6. Giraudet-LeQuintrec JS and others: Positive effect of patient education for hip surgery, *Clin Orthopaed Rel Re*s 414:112-120, 2003.

7. Glass C, Grap MJ, Battle G: Preparing the patient and family for home mechanical ventilation, *Med Surg Nurs* 8:99-107, 1999.

8. Gray MJ, Elhai JD, Frueh BC: Enhancing patient satisfaction and increasing treatment compliance: patient education as a fundamental component of PTSD treatment, *Psychiatr Q* 75:321-332, 2004.

9. Hammond A, Freeman K: The long-term outcomes from a randomized controlled trial of an educational-behavioural joint protection programme for people with rheumatoid arthritis, *Clin Rehabil* 18:520-528, 2004.

10. Heitkemper MM and others: Self-management for women with irritable bowel syndrome, *Clin Gastroenterol Hepatol* 2:585-596, 2004.

11. Hering K, Harvan J, D'Angelo M, Jasinski D: The use of a computer website prior to scheduled surgery (a pilot study): Impact on patient information, acquisition, anxiety level, and overall satisfaction with anesthesia care, *AANA J* 73:29-33, 2005.

12. Knoerl D and others: Preoperative PCA teaching program to manage postoperative pain, *Med Surg Nurs* 8:25-33, 36, 1999.

13. Kulp JL, Rane S, Bachmann G: Impact of preventive osteoporosis education on patient behavior: Immediate and 3-month follow-up, *Menopause* 11:116-119, 2004.

14. Landsvert SS, Kane CR: Antonovsky's sense of coherence: theoretical basis of psychoeducation in schizophrenia, *Issues Ment Health Nurs* 19:419-431, 1998.

15. Lorig KR, Ritter PL, Laurent DD, Fries JF: Long-term randomized controlled trials of tailored-print and small-group arthritis self-management interventions, *Med Care* 42:346-354, 2004.

16. Lorig K and others: Arthritis self-management program variations: three studies, *Arthritis Care Res* 11:448-454, 1998.

17. McFarlane WR, Dixon L, Lukens E, Lucksted A: Family psychoeducation and schizophrenia: a review of the literature, *J Marital Fam Ther* 29:223-245, 2003.

18. McGregor AH, Rylands H, Owen A, Dore CJ, Hughes SPF: Does preoperative hip rehabilitation advice improve recovery and patient satisfaction? *J Arthroplasty* 19:464-468, 2004.

19. Niedermann K, Fransen J, Knols R, Uebelhart D: Gap between short- and long-term effects of patients education in rheumatoid arthritis patients: A systematic review, *Arthritis Care Res* 51:388-398, 2004.

20. Perry A and others: Randomised controlled trial of efficacy of teaching patients with bipolar disorder to identify early symptoms of relapse and obtain treatment, *BMJ* 318:149-153, 1999.

21. Reinares M and others: Impact of a psychoeducational family intervention on caregivers of stabilized bipolar patients, *Psychother Psychosom* 73:312-319, 2004.

22. Riemsma RP, Taal E, Kirwan JR, Rasker JJ: Systematic review of rheumatoid arthritis patient education, *Arthritis Care Res* 51:1045-1059, 2004.

23. Subak LL, Quesenberry CP, Posner SF, Cattolica E, Soghikian K: The effect of behavioral therapy on urinary incontinence: A randomized controlled trial, *Obstet Gynecol* 100:72-78, 2002.

24. Warsi A, LaVelley MP, Wang PS, Avorn J, Solomon DH: Arthritis self-management education programs, *Arthritis Rheum* 48:2207-2213, 2003.

25. Wholihan D: A patient education tool for patient-controlled analgesia, *Oncol Nurs Forum* 24:1801-1804, 1997.

26. Wong AL, Harker JO, Lau VP, Shatzel S, Port LH: Spanish arthritis empowerment program: A dissemination and effectiveness study, *Arthritis Care Res* 51:332-336, 2004.

9

Patient Education Delivery, Health Policy, and New Directions

DELIVERY OF PATIENT EDUCATION

Patient education is currently defined as an essential part of practice in state practice acts for most health professionals, in various federal and state regulations, and in accreditation criteria. Because patient education has not usually been a reimbursable service and thus does not bring in revenue, the degree of formalization of a structure for delivery of these services seems to have fluctuated and may now be at a lower ebb than it was during the 1980s.

Nettles's[19] review of the evolution of diabetes education depicts delivery changes. From 1950 to 1970, persons with diabetes (especially type 1) were admitted to hospitals. Given that there would be a long stay, nurses along with inpatient dietitians provided one-to-one instruction with multiple opportunities for patient practice. Group classes were rare in this setting, and outpatient programs were not usually available. Now, if newly diagnosed persons with diabetes are hospitalized, they have short lengths of stay with limited time for instruction. Referral to home health agencies for continued instruction has become more common.

Diabetes education has now been expanded to incorporate comorbidities and complications.

The health care system in the United States still contains significant managed care and capitated arrangements. This situation creates more positive incentives to use education to teach people how to manage their own self-care and avoid the use of expensive institutional services. In spite of these changed incentives, it is not clear how many patients who are in need of appropriate patient education actually receive it. Apparently no data about the availablility of patient education services in nonhospital sectors of the health care industry are available.

Very limited data are available about patient education services. In 1999 the American Hospital Association reported that 52% of hospitals in the United States have a patient education center and 40% a health information center,[1] more likely to be offered in institutions not under governmental control and not for profit, in larger and urban hospitals and those in networks.[20]

Large surveys of patients' perceptions of their experiences in hospitals show a significant lack

of satisfaction with the educational and supportive aspects of care. Many patients believed
hospitals did not do well at providing emotional
support and alleviating fears and anxieties or
in preparing patients to go home. They saw a
confusing, expensive, unreliable, and often im-
personal disassembly of health professionals and
institutions. Patients talk about how assertive
they must be to get answers and the frustrations
of trying to coordinate care among many different
specialists. About one third of hospital patients
indicated that they had not been told about
danger signals to watch for after they went home,
side effects of medicines they were to take, or
when they could expect to resume normal activities or that they did not have a say regarding
their treatment. Patients often expressed the fear
that information about their illness or prognosis
was being withheld from them.[2]

Several kinds of initiatives in which patient
education is central can be cited.

- Patient learning centers are sometimes
  available in health care institutions. The
  center is a laboratory-like environment for
  learning, practicing, and demonstrating self-
  care skills such as blood pressure and pulse
  monitoring, self-administration of insulin
  and monitoring blood glucose, breast-
  feeding, well newborn care, and caring for a
  person recovering at home. Many centers
  focus as well on building self-efficacy among
  patients and their families for managing
  their own care. Insurance companies may
  cover the fees charged for use of the patient
  learning center.[10,16]

- Nurse-managed clinics providing self-care
  education are useful for many diseases.
  Lorig and others[18] have shown that it is
  possible to teach patients with a variety of
  chronic illnesses (heart or lung disease,
  stroke, or arthritis) in one group. Common
  self-management skills that need to be
  learned include recognizing and acting on
  symptoms, using medications correctly,
  managing emergencies, maintaining nutrition
  and diet and adequate exercise, using stress
  reduction techniques, interacting effectively
  with health care providers, managing relation-

ships with significant others, adapting to
work, and managing psychological responses
to illness, such as depression.

- New roles, such as renal patient educator,
  are evolving to meet education and triaging
  functions across phases of the disease and
  settings in which care is provided. For
  example, faced with an intake of 280 new
  renal patients from six area hospitals plus
  private practice, the need to educate patients
  regarding treatment modalities and selection
  and to triage patients into 10 of its own plus
  other dialysis facilities, a clinic in central
  Missouri has relied on the role of a dialysis
  patient educator. The educator's role
  involves contacting and assessing new renal
  patients and families and providing one-
  on-one and small group education about
  endstage renal disease and treament options
  in a neutral manner. Emphasis is placed on
  both technical aspects and the advantages
  and disadvantages of each for patients' lifestyles, medical histories, and needs. Education sessions usually range from 30 to 90
  minutes in length. Dialysis and transplant
  nurses refer to the educator if patients are in
  need of education concerning changing a
  treatment modality.[5]

- Sometimes the specialist nurses in these
  roles provide patient education and clinical
  recommendations for general practitioners
  and practice nurses as well as direct clinical
  support for patients (often called a liaison
  model). With use of such a practice role,
  unscheduled care for acute asthma in a poor
  population was reduced despite comparison
  with a control group of practices receiving
  educational outreach for asthma, which itself
  improves care.[11] In a similar role, working
  with both providers and high health care
  user patients, asthma nurse specialists
  suggested to the primary care physician
  potential simplilfication or consolidation of
  patients' current regimens; provided asthma
  education appropriate to the patients' education, motivation and cultural beliefs; provided
  psychosocial support and screened patient
  need for professional counseling; developed

individualized asthma self-management plans; facilitated discharge planning; and provided outpatient follow-up through phone contact, home visits, and appointments with the primary care physician as necessary. In this randomized controlled trial, expensive hospitalizations were reduced by 54% versus 42% in the control group.[6]

Others have used hospital or community-based systems structures. In some instances the system consists of hospital staff nurses serving as unit patient educators, free patient education television channels, reference books of patient education plans on each unit, an interdisciplinary patient/family education committee, and a Web site with low-literacy patient education materials.[7] A neighborhood asthma coalition instituted a promotional and educational campaign, encouraging involvement of residents in planning and implementing asthma management classes and providing social support for parents and children with asthma. Although those with regular contact with the program showed a significant reduction in the acute asthma care rate, only 19% of the intervention group demonstrated this level of interaction with program staff.[9]

Other approaches link mainstream health care facilities with specialized educational centers. For example, a managed-care organization outsourced diabetes education services to a free-standing, community-based diabetes disease state management center staffed by practicing certified diabetes educators, who counsel and instruct patients in every aspect of diabetes treatment. Primary care physicians in managed-care organizations were found not to have time to work with patients on diabetes self-management skills. The specialized educational center achieved a 72% decrease in hospital stays, 71% fewer emergency department (ED) visits, and a 63% drop in missed work days.[12] In the 1990s, the province of Quebec established more than a hundred asthma education centers. Because only a small proportion of patients were sent to these centers, one hospital with a high rate of ED visits by these patients provided a short intervention of teaching inhaler technique and use of an action plan and made an automatic referral to an asthma education center. In only

4 months the number of patients referred for formal asthma education increased more than tenfold and ED visits dropped.[22]

IMPORTANT POLICY ISSUES

Policies about who is to do patient education and whether and how it is paid for are important. A 1990 federal law and subsequent state laws require pharmacists to provide counseling about prescription drugs. A recent study of 306 community pharmacies in eight states found that the counseling received by trained shoppers (acting as patients) varied significantly, with frequency climbing from 40% to 94% as states' counseling regulations increased in frequency. Busyness and recency of pharmacist training also predicted the amount of patient counseling. Some states require counseling for all patients, performed personally and face to face by a pharmacist. In contrast, other states require only an "offer to counsel" made by licensed or nonlicensed personnel. In this study, 47% of all shoppers never received any oral drug information from pharmacy staff when they presented three prescriptions.[23]

Lack of insurance payment for patient education has long been a barrier to its provision. Services that reduce errors such as anticoagulation clinics operated by nurses or patient counseling by retail pharmacists are frequently not reimbursed, whereas care that is unsafe is paid for and physicians and hospitals can bill for the additional services that are needed when patients are injured by their mistakes.[17] Best developed are policies by more than 30 states that mandate coverage of diabetes education and supplies and Medicare reimbursement for non-hospital-based educational and training services and blood glucose monitoring supplies.[12] An estimate of the size of the unreimbursed cost of patient education provided by nurses in a large medical group practice and associated hospitals ranged from $28 to $49 million annually. Yet patient education is believed to be essential to good practice.[25] Estimates of the intensity and length of patient education (and thus its cost) for various groups are generally not available. Brown and others'[4] study of diabetes education for poor Mexican-Americans with very elevated glucose levels showed a clear dosage effect; attending more sessions resulted in greater improvements in metabolic control. Typical diabetes education programs range from 4 to 15 hours over a 2- to 3-month period and cost between $95 and $125 per 1-hour session; group instruction costs slightly less. Effective education in the study of Brown and others[4] took 52 hours over a 12-month period. Costs were reduced by offering group instruction in free community sites.

In general, the value of pharmaceuticals is much more accepted, unquestioned, and reimbursed than is that of patient education services. Nurse-led outpatient management including education for groups such as those with child-hood asthma have been shown to be more cost-effective than pediatrician care. This substitution offers a cost-effective way to obtain the kinds of patient outcomes that can be produced by education, also reaping the commonly demonstrated savings in hospitalization and ED visits.[15]

NEW AREAS OF PATIENT EDUCATION

Most patient education must incorporate methods that are known to change behavior. A variety of behavioral change models are available to guide interventions. Clear guidelines for their use may be found in Box 9-1.[18] (Most have been reviewed in previous chapters.)

Clearly, the most rapidly developing area of patient education practice is self-management,

---

| Box 9-1 | *Guidelines for Provider Counseling Actions as Suggested by Health Behavior Change Theories* |

1. Cognition and Information-Processing Models

Assess the extent to which the patient has thought about the issues and how much information he or she has previously received on the topic.

Present information based on patient's previous experience with the behavior change.

Stress important information first.

Provide both sensory and procedural information.

Provide written information based on the patient's educational level.

Check for comprehension of material and fit with previous schema.

2. Health Belief Model

Assess the patient's perceived susceptibility and severity of the outcome and frame the health message according to these perceptions.

Elicit perceived barriers to the health-behavior change in question and discuss how to overcome these barriers.

Assess the perceived benefits for engaging in the behavior and incorporate these benefits as reinforcers for behavior.

3. Theory of Reasoned Action

Determine whether the patient thinks family members and friends endorse the behavior.

Highlight the social pressure to engage in the behavior if it exists.

Provide examples of similar others who are currently engaging in the behavior.

Use specific examples of behaviors when assessing behavioral intentions.

4. Social Cognitive Theory

Increase self-efficacy for the behavior.

Provide opportunities for the patient to master the necessary skills.

Model or provide models of the targeted behavior.

Ask the patient to rehearse the behavior and provide feedback on his or her performance.

Address previously failed attempts and explore individual and environmental factors that may have contributed to these unsuccessful attempts.

Explore successes with other health behavior changes and techniques used that may generalize to the targeted behavior change.

Increase outcome expectancies for the behavior.

From Elder JP, Ayala GX, Harris S: Theories and intervention approaches to health-behavior change in primary care, *Am J Prev Med* 17:275-284, 1999.

Box 9-1	*Guidelines for Provider Counseling Actions as Suggested by Health Behavior Change Theories—*cont'd

Provide information to the patient on the efficacy of the behavior.

Arrange for the patient to meet a similar other who has experience with the behavior and endorses its effectiveness.

5. Behavior Modification

Determine whether a skill or performance deficit exists.

Teach the patient the necessary skills to engage in the behavior.

Reduce punishment for pro-health behavior.

Reduce reinforcement for health-damaging behavior.

Agree on positive reinforcers to be used as behavior change occurs.

Agree on negative reinforcers to be used when behavior change does not occur.

Reinforce the behavior by inquiring about its performance.

6. Self-Management

Teach the patient how to monitor his or her own behavior.

Help the patient to become aware of internal cues for the behavior he or she is attempting to extinguish.

Decide on alternative, competing behaviors in which the patient can engage.

Identify, with the patient, external cues for the behavior.

Teach the patient how to use external cues to reinforce appropriate behavior or strategies to reduce the likelihood of engaging in inappropriate behavior.

7. Interpersonal and Social-Support Theories

Convey empathy and understanding for the difficulties of behavior change.

Provide a private setting in which to repeat and clarify instructions and assess resistance to change.

Schedule follow-up visits to evaluate the patient's progress and demonstrate commitment to provide support during the change process.

Engage the family in the targeted behavior.

Address the entire family to gain commitment from all members for support of the behavior change.

8. Transtheoretical Model

Assess the patient's stage of change by minimally assessing whether he or she is currently engaging in the behavior or whether he or she has thought about possible changes to improve his or her health. Use motivational interviewing techniques such as expressing empathy, providing a menu of options, and avoiding argumentation.

Persons in the precontemplation stage should be made aware of the consequences for not engaging in health-behavior change, be provided the opportunity to share their feelings about their condition and discuss how their behavior affects the rest of the family.

People who are contemplators should be taught to closely monitor their motivations for engaging in the health-behavior change and explore their ambivalence and reasons they think change might be beneficial.

Individuals in the preparation stage should be asked to verbalize a commitment to change both to themselves and to their family members.

Action-stage individuals and those in the maintenance stage should work with the provider to set up rewards for appropriate behavior and stress-management techniques and establish supportive relationships.

From Elder JP, Ayala GX, Harris S: Theories and intervention approaches to health-behavior change in primary care, *Am J Prev Med* 17:275-284, 1999.

representing both an economic and a philosophical shift.

- The number of self-tests continues to increase. Figure 9-1 provides brief information about a self-test for chlamydia. Vaginal introital specimens are self-collected with use of only an instructional booklet.[21]

- A pilot study suggests that oncology patients and participants in clinical trials can submit treatment toxicity information directly through a Web-based patient-reporting system. As patients experience adverse effects, their needs for therapy modifications, supportive care, and education often change; constant patient reporting monitored by health professionals allows a timely response. Traditionally, patients have been viewed as being incapable of directly reporting their symptoms, and a model has evolved in which patient experiences are elicited, filtered, and reported by health care professionals.[3]

- A new kind of information booklet for patients with chronic arthritis is patient generated and contains the illness narratives of patients with three kinds of arthritis. The booklet draws on the knowledge of patients who feel they are flourishing despite their condition. Instructive narratives are grounded in experience and enforce reflection, are memorable, and foster empathy and construction of meaning around the illness. Reading about others' feelings can give a person "permission" to feel the same emotions, and those who lack social support can

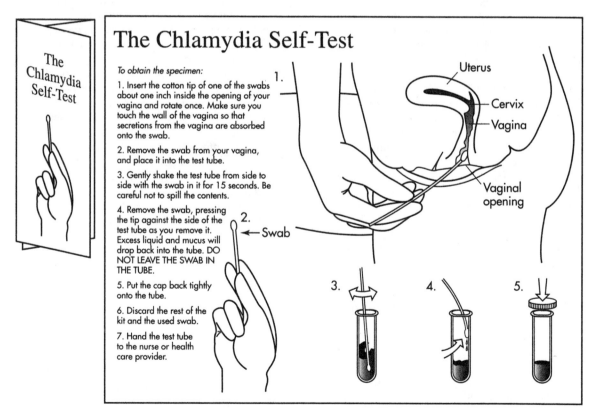

FIGURE 9-1   Polymerase chain reaction self-test instruction booklet used in this study. (From Polaneczky M and others: Use of self-collected vaginal specimens for detection of *Chlamydia trachomatis* infection, *Obstet Gynecol* 91:375-378, 1998.)

feel supported. The United Kingdom's National Health Service defines expert patients as "people living with a long-term health condition, who are able to take more control over their health by understanding and managing their conditions, leading to an improved quality of life."[24]

- Screening has frequently been promoted as a beneficial, preventive activity that all eligible people should participate in for the good of the whole, although some people will inevitably be harmed. The United Kingdom now has policies in place that require health

professionals to ensure that individuals are making an individual informed choice about being screened, a shift from a predominantly utilitarian philosophy to a liberal one.[14] Indeed, evidence-based patient choice is defined as offering patients research-based information and the opportunity to influence decisions about their treatment and care. Tables 9-1 and 9-2 provide patient decision templates for treatment options and for screening options. The preferred style of the clinical encounter is widely assumed to have moved from paternalism to partner-

TABLE 9-1   **Patient Decision Template for Treatment Options**

Required Element	Key Patient Questions	Information Provided
Clinical condition reported	What are the characteristics of my diagnosis/disease/disorder?	Details of clinically important subgroups
Patient decision situation	What are the different ways this disorder can be treated?	Options for surgical treatments, medical treatments, watchful waiting, complementary therapies
For each treatment option:		
Treatment processes	What kind of treatment is it? How much time does it involve? What do I have to do to undergo this treatment?	Mode and duration of treatment, nature of patient involvement
Outcomes and probabilities	What are the chances of improvement over the next x days/weeks/months/years or over my lifetime?	Rates for different outcomes over various times, absolute number improved, improvement rate
	What kinds of side/toxic effects can happen, and what are the chances of each?	Rates for different side effects
Value tradeoffs	What are the tradeoffs between length of life and quality of life? If length of life is not affected, what are the tradeoffs among the inconveniences, costs, chances of side effects, etc, in order to gain a benefit like symptom relief?	Material for clarification of values
	Where can I get descriptions of other patients' experiences?	

From Holmes-Rovner M and others: Patient choice modules for summaries of clinical effectiveness: A proposal, *Br Med J* 322:664-667, 2001. Reproduced with permission from the BMJ Publishing Group.

TABLE 9-2	**Patient Decision Template for Screening Options**	
Required Element	**Key Patient Questions**	**Information Provided**
Clinical condition to be prevented	What are the characteristics of this diagnosis/disease/disorder?	Expected incidence of disease in 1, 5, 10, and 20 years among untreated patients Identification of clinically important subgroups at risk Probabilities of key patient-oriented outcomes (harms and benefits) caused by the disease if untreated
Patient decision situation	What are the different ways this disease/disorder can be detected/prevented?	Options in terms of screening, watchful waiting, medical preventive strategies, lifestyle preventive strategies
Effectiveness of treatment if detected by screening	If the disease/disorder is detected by screening, how effective is the subsequent treatment?	Probabilities of key patient-oriented harms and benefits, in terms of difference from rates in unscreened population Absolute risk reduction Relative risk reduction
Screening options (for each possible test)	What are the side effects of taking this test?	Rates of side effects
	How accurate is this test?	Rates for false positive and negative results
	What happens after I take the test?	Follow-up procedures
Value tradeoffs	Am I willing to go through the potential anxiety of screening and treatment now to prevent a disease in the future?	
	What impact will screening have on my family and professional life?	Material for clarification of values

From Holmes-Rovner M and others: Patient choice modules for summaries of clinical effectiveness: A proposal, *Br Med J* 322:664-667, 2001. Reproduced with permission from the BMJ Publishing Group.

ship, requiring patients to be well informed and able to make their own decisions.[13]

SUMMARY

Although a number of innovative delivery systems for patient education have been documented, they are not comprehensive enough or sufficiently supported by payment policies to ensure anywhere near sufficient availability. A strong move toward self-management education is evident.

REFERENCES

1. American Hospital Association: *Hospital statistics.* Chicago, 1999, The Association.

2. American Hospital Association, Picker Institute: Eye on patients: Excerpts from a report on patients' concerns and experiences about the health care system, *J Health Care Finance* 2:2-11, 1997.

3. Basch E and others: Patient online self-reporting of toxicity symptoms during chemotherapy, *J Clin Oncol* 23:3552-3561, 2005.

4. Brown S and others: Dosage effects of diabetes self-management education for Mexican-Americans, *Diabetes Care* 28:527-532, 2005.

5. Campbell A: Improvement of patient care through a collaborative approach to patient education and triage, *AdvRenal Replac Ther* 6:347-350, 1999.

6. Castro M and others: Asthma intervention program prevents readmissions in high healthcare users, *Am J Respir Crit Care Med* 168:1095-1099, 2003.

7. Duffy ML: Designing a comprehensive hospital-wide patient education program, *Adv Renal Replac Ther* 6:289-293, 1999.

8. Elder JP, Ayala GX, Harris S: Theories and intervention approaches to health-behavior change in primary care, *Am J Prev Med* 17:275-284, 1999.

9. Fisher ED and others: Community organization to reduce the need for acute care for asthma among African American children in low-income neighborhoods: The Neighborhood Asthma Coalition, *Pediatrics* 114:116-123, 2004.

10. Goldstein NL and others: Comparison of two teaching strategies, *Clin Nurs Res* 5:150-166, 1996.

11. Griffiths C and others: Specialist nurse intervention to reduce unscheduled asthma care in a deprived multiethnic area: The east London randomised controlled trial for high risk asthma (ELECTRA), *BMJ* 328:144-147, 2004.

12. Hendricks LE, Hendricks RT: Making a case for the CDE's role in outsourcing diabetes services to a freestanding outpatient diabetes disease state management center, *Diabetes Educ* 25:766-773, 1999.

13. Holmes-Rovner M and others: Patient choice modules for summaries of clinical effectiveness: A proposal, *BMJ* 322:664-667, 2001.

14. Jepson RG, Hewison J, Thompson AGH, Weller D: How should we measure informed choice? The case of cancer screening, *J Med Ethics* 31:192-196, 2005.

15. Kamps AWA and others: Impact of nurse-led outpatient management of children with asthma on healthcare resource utilisation and costs, *Eur Respir J* 23:304-309, 2004.

16. Kantz B and others: Developing patient and family education services, *J Nurs Adm* 28:11-18, 1998.

17. Leape LL, Berwick DM: Five years after To Err Is Human: What have we learned? *JAMA* 293:2384-2390, 2005.

18. Lorig KR and others: Evidence suggesting that a chronic disease self-management program can improve health status while reducing hospitalization, *Med Care* 37:5-14, 1999.

19. Nettles AT: Patient education in the hospital, *Diabetes Spectrum* 18:44-48, 2005.

20. Olden PC, Clement DG: The prevalence of hospital health promotion and disease prevention services: Good news, bad news and policy implications, *Milbank Q* 78:115-146, 2000.

21. Polaneczky M and others: Use of self-collected vaginal specimens for detection of *Chlamydia trachomatis* infection, *Obstet Gynecol* 91:375-378, 1998.

22. Robichaud P and others: Evaluation of a program aimed at increasing referrals for asthma education of patients consulting at the emergency department for acute care, *Chest* 126:1495-1501, 2004.

23. Svarstad BL, Bultman DC, Mount JK: Patient counseling provided in community pharmacies: Effects of state regulation, pharmacist age, and busyness, *J Am Pharm Assoc* 44:22-29, 2004.

24. Swift TL, Dieppe PA: Using expert patients' narratives as an educational resource, *Patient Educ Couns* 57:115-121, 2005.

25. Williams AR and others: Estimation of unreimbursed patient education costs at a large group practice, *J Contin Educ Health Prof* 24:12-19, 2004.

Suggested Answers to Study Questions

1. The implications are that all encounters with the health care system must advance patients' understanding so that they can better manage their own health.
2. Evidence of wanting to learn is important for situations a and b.
   a. Your questions should determine the women's understanding and feelings about cancer, about preventive care in general, about manipulating their own breasts, and about the meaning of finding a lump. Some may have had instruction in the procedure and will be able to do some or all of it correctly.
   b. Some of your questions should enable you to discover the level of disability the boy is experiencing. Can he understand language and, if so, which words? How well can he grasp things and move his arms in a feeling motion? Other questions will deal with his independence and his caregiver's ability to cooperate in the training program. Does everyone in the family (including the boy) want the child to be independent? Is the caregiver patient yet precise enough to carry out a training program? Could she interpret the boy's behavior in terms of progress toward the goal?
3. You should not be surprised by these findings: they are what you would expect given an understanding of learning theory. Among the learning principles involved are that practice improves memory, direct experience of the skill helps the parent retain more learning than does an abstract review, and successful experience with feedback increases self-efficacy for that skill.
4. a. Establishing baseline.
   b. Modeling.
   c. Setting up reinforcement; however, it would be useful to know if giving pennies for toys reinforces the child's behavior.
   d. Shaping.
   e. Contingent reinforcement.

CHAPTER 2: EDUCATIONAL OBJECTIVES AND INSTRUCTION

1. No, because the implicit (although never stated) objectives of discharge care involve observing the wound for evidence of complications, which requires being able to recognize such signs and symptoms.
2. The nurse can suggest that the mother place green peas, cereal bits, apple slices, and other similar foods on the baby's food tray to provide practice of skills he or she needs to develop. Explanation of the organizing idea should also be given to the mother to show ways in which she can aid the baby's development. The U.S. Department of Agriculture has simple large-print booklets on this subject that can be read by mothers with limited literacy. The nurse can directly facilitate learning through modeling play and vocal games with the infant during visits and through his or her own expression of pleasure. All three of these strategies can be used. If this learning goal is needed by a number of mothers, consider developing a group teaching situation.

CHAPTER 3: EVALUATION IN PATIENT EDUCATION

1. To comprehend the means of attaining asepsis in giving an injection.
2. Transfer is involved every time the evaluation task is different from the learning tasks. Such is the case with all levels of complexity with the possible exception of knowledge (cognitive). It is possible to index the degree of transfer of which the learner is capable by systematic testing of a variety of situations that require varying degrees of transfer (on a continuum from those tasks that are very much like the original learning task to those that are very little like it).
3. Factors and action (see below):

Possible Factors Causing Inattentiveness and Rebelliousness	Nurse Action
The complexity of the task the nurse was teaching might have been too great for the learner's ability, resulting in failure or even lack of willingness to begin learning.	Do a more careful analysis of prerequisite skills the learner possesses. If the goals are found to be too complex, break the skills into smaller units or teach the last part of the skill first (so that the learner experiences success).
The individual may be preoccupied with other life problems and therefore may not feel motivated to develop this new behavior.	Assess the accuracy of this hypothesis by talking with the learner and others who know him and by watching his behavior. It may be possible to create motivation by persuading him that learning the dressing skills can help him solve the other problem. Another alternative is to wait a few weeks and try again.
This may be the individual's usual response to many things.	Assess the validity of this statement. If true, it may be possible to do some teaching in spite of the inattentiveness and rebelliousness. The success of learning may alter these responses. Another alternative is teaching aimed first at altering these attitudes.

4. Analyzing patient's understanding:
    a. This person may not understand how blood sugar is measured—a certain amount per standard volume of blood. Investigate this.
    b. This is likely to be indicative of affective rather than cognitive learning. Because the patient is in the somewhat ambiguous situation of not being insulin dependent, she is not motivated to move beyond the lower levels of the affective domain. It is also possible that she has not progressed beyond the denial or disbelief stage of psychosocial adaptation to illness.
    c. This comment may be evaluative of either cognitive objectives or affective objectives or both. See whether the rest of the conversation provides a more specific clue, and, if not, question the father yourself. The comment may mean that the man has not understood how diabetic patients accommodate activities such as hunting trips, or it may represent a seeking of verification from an experienced person that diabetic patients really can hunt and that his son can participate in such physically taxing activities.
5. The evaluation approach is very appropriate because these behaviors and clinical thinking are crucial to the patient's well-being. The reason this approach is very infrequently used is that it is expensive of time and materials. The evaluative judgment made as a result of the objective structured clinical examination is likely to be highly accurate.

CHAPTER 4: CANCER PATIENT EDUCATION

1. The critique should include (1) whether the questions test crucial elements, especially those that are commonly misunderstood by this population, (2) whether the reading level is so high that patients cannot understand the questions, (3) whether the score would represent true knowledge, and (4) whether the objective of increasing knowledge about screening will really contribute to any important clinical objective. My judgment is that the test is flawed on each of these criteria.

2. Not likely. What you probably want to know is how women examine their breasts (have them demonstrate) and if men can draw or describe where their prostate gland is. The questions as they are currently worded will not provide this most important information.
3. From a medical perspective it seems thorough. It does not include behavioral outcomes—only topics to be taught—and there is no evidence that it represents what patients need to know.
4. It is likely too verbal—not sufficiently pictorial. At best it could be used as a reminder of the demonstration and a focus for practice to a level of confidence witnn use of silicone models and real breasts.
5. There is evidence that chemotherapy is associated with these problems.

CHAPTER 7: EDUCATION FOR PREGNANCY AND PARENTING AND EDUCATION OF CHILDREN

1. Practice to overlearning; assessment and feedback from instructor and further instruction if necessary; speaking with parents who have used these skills successfully (modeling); and at least yearly re-education to maintain skills.
2. Clearly the development of self-efficacy could be one framework within which to view this interaction. Early in the vignette the mother lacked self-efficacy but gained it as she had real life experience under the coaching of the nurse. Remember how empowering self-efficacy can be; it focuses and motivates behavior. One could also use a physiological/ developmental learning framework on the part of the infant, and one could use the process of parent-infant attachment as a framework.
3. It would be useful to have observational evidence that what parents report is what they actually do. It would also be useful to understand sources of disagreement further before labeling these populations as noncompliant and to check their sense of efficacy in carrying out these recommendations. Community-based interventions with parents who have

had experience with this issue are likely to be persuasive. In the end, parents will make their own decisions.

SUGGESTED ANSWERS TO CASE QUESTIONS

NOTE: Not all cases include questions.

Chapter 4: Cancer Patient Eduction

Case I: There are two presumed patient objectives: (1) to describe the sequence of catheter care and (2) to safely provide catheter care in the home with a low infection rate. You need to test the patients and families to see if these objectives have been met—highly doubtful. Demonstration is the correct teaching approach for the second objective, but it's flawed because patients could not see the torso model and, more importantly, did not return the demonstration and receive feedback. The appropriate approach is for each patient to return the demonstration until it is done correctly and the patient is confident. Do patients know what an infection looks like?

Case II: Assessing needs of actual patients and then getting feedback on the PIL from similar women before its use increases the likelihood of its being valid. Assume that some other method will be used for women of low literacy. The objectives are incorrectly written—they address what teachers should do, not patients, which leaves in question criteria on which the PIL's evaluation will be based.

Chapter 5: Cardiovascular and Pulmonary Patient Education

Case I: These findings could be explained by lack of payment and incentives for delivering this care and lack of holding providers accountable for doing so. Unfortunately, this pattern is widely descriptive of patient education/self-management for chronic diseases in the United States.

Case II: A) Not surprised including about academic hospitals because they are the strongest bastions of medical model practice. B) The quickest way to resolve the problem is not to pay for the care of these patients unless discharge education is properly done to standard. The justification for such an action is that patients are being harmed by this substandard practice, clearly a violation of professional ethics.

Chapter 6: Diabetes Self-Management Education

Case I: You would not let him sit silently during the whole class. A preassessment for each patient (before the formal class) should check for literacy (which fits the pattern of consistently not being able to find the right page) as well as readiness to learn.

Chapter 7: Education for Pregnancy and Parenting and Educating Children

Case I: Feminists would say this represents a bias characteristic of medical and societal views about pronatalist motherhood and women being valued primarily as receptacles for babies. Because the mother's personal needs and her lack of confidence in caring for her baby, feminists would say this is an example of unethical teaching. Another perspective would note how difficult it is to obtain realistic learning experiences postpartum because women are isolated in their homes. But prenatal education could build appropriate expectations, problem solving, and coping skills specifically oriented to the postpartum time, support groups, and warm lines for nursing advice and teaching.

Additional Study Aids

ADDITIONAL STUDY QUESTIONS AND ANSWERS

1. A radiology department found a problem of excessive repeat rates on some of its x-ray series, often because of poor bowel preparation. How would you justify development of a patient education program on preparation for these tests? What level of success could you promise?

2. Researchers in diabetes have found that self-care behaviors are often only weakly correlated with glycemic control.[6] What is the relevance of this finding for learning?

3. Studies show that feelings of control are important to psychosocial recovery from a cardiac event[10] and that disease severity is not a reliable predictor of psychosocial recovery. This is also true for other illnesses such as cancer and rheumatoid arthritis. Perceptions of control are associated with increased adherence in persons with diabetes, patients undergoing cardiac rehabilitation, and individuals with hypertension. How can patient education be designed to develop perceived control by patients?

4. Preparing patients to play a major role in choice of treatments is a goal of patient education. Some of the most structured work toward this goal has been done for persons choosing treatment for benign prostatic hypertrophy. Box 1 contains symptom questions and value questions that reflect the patient's perspective and thus help him make a treatment decision.[1] Construct a similar set of symptom and value questions for helping patients with another disorder make a treatment decision.

5. In Box 2, match the theory most identified with the following teaching approaches (theories may be used more than once).

6. Recent research using qualitative methods shows that individuals use biomedical information selectively and incorporate it into their own experiences and sources of information, to make it "their own."

   a. What philosophy of learning best describes this process?

| Box 1 | *Symptom and Value Questions* |

Symptom Questions

Over the past month or so, how often have you:

1. Had a burning feeling when you urinate?
2. Had to push or strain to begin urination?
3. Had to urinate again shortly after you were finished urinating?
4. Found you stopped and started again several times when you urinated?
5. Dribbled urine after you thought you were finished urinating?
6. Ordered categorical responses: (1) not at all, (2) a few times, (3) fairly often, (4) usually, (5) always.

Value Questions

1. Suppose your urinary symptoms stayed just the same as they are now for the rest of your life. How would you feel about that?

2. Suppose a treatment cured your urinary symptoms, but after the treatment any sexual climaxes would result in retrograde ejaculation. How would you feel about your situation?
3. Suppose a treatment cured your urinary symptoms, but you were not able to have sexual erections. How would you feel about your situation?
4. Suppose a treatment cured your urinary symptoms, but you occasionally dripped urine or wet your pants slightly. How would you feel about your situation?

Ordered categorical responses: (1) delighted, (2) pleased, (3) mostly satisfied, (4) mixed, (5) mostly dissatisfied, (6) unhappy, (7) terrible.

From Barry MJ and others: Patient reactions to a program designed to facilitate patient participation in treatment decisions for benign prostatic hyperplasia, *Med Care* 33:771-782, 1995.

| Box 2 | *Teaching Approaches and Theories* |

Teaching Approaches

1. Emphasis on seriousness of consequences of not taking a health action
2. Consciousness raising
3. Reinterpretation of physiological signs and symptoms
4. Relapse prevention
5. Modeling
6. Provision of cues to precipitate action

Theories

a. Self-efficacy theory

b. Transtheoretical model of change
c. Health belief model

Circle the correct answer
T F 7. A health care provider may be sued for a negative event resulting from the patient not understanding discharge instructions.
T F 8. Traditionally the goal of patient education has been compliance with the medical regimen.

b. What does this philosophy predict about the quality of learning that comes from such a process?
c. How should health professionals respond to such knowledge?

7. Piette and others[11] described a study of automated telephone assessment and self-care education with nurse follow-up to persons with diabetes. During biweekly 5- to 8-minute telephone assessments, patients interacted

with the system using their touch-tone keypad; responses were stored and determined the subsequent content of the message. During each assessment, patients reported information about self-monitored blood glucose readings, self-care, perceived glycemic control, and symptoms of poor glycemic control, foot problems, chest pain, and breathing problems. Patients also heard educational messages focusing on glucose self-monitoring, foot care, and medication adherence; reported specific barriers to self-care; and received tailored messages and advice. Each week, the automated assessment system generated reports organized according to the urgency of reported problems, and the nurse used these reports to prioritize patient contacts. On average, patients had 6 minutes of nurse telephone contact per month. In comparison with the usual-care group, these patients had improved self-care and glycemic control and decreased symptom burden.

Identify two elements of the intervention with good potential to create learning, including change in behavior.

8. It is estimated that 21% of the adult population in the United States has only rudimentary reading and writing skills. A recent study of patients on warfarin therapy showed that those with a lower numeracy level spent more time with warfarin levels above their therapeutic ranges. Time spent in range has been directly associated with bleeding complications. Warfarin therapy requires frequent monitoring, dose adjustment, and an ability to follow instructions very closely. Patients are often instructed to cut tablets in half, to take different daily doses, or to use different tablet strengths.[5] Are you surprised by the study's findings? What can you do to increase safety for these patients?

9. In a randomized controlled trial, diabetics discharged early and receiving follow-up phone calls from a nurse did better (lower HbA_{1c}) at 24 weeks than did those who continued to receive routine hospital care.[12] What could account for these findings?

10. Young Teen Asthma Camp (ages 12-15 years) had the following goals:

"To provide an experience in camping for teens with asthma that supports a positive identity, creates opportunities for learning new skills, and creates a nurturing environment for teen development.

To provide opportunity for education on asthma self-care and support service utilization for teens with asthma.

To provide opportunities for social development and friendships among teens of similar ages to enhance resilience and effective coping with asthma."[3]

The camp setting provides the very environment in which exposure to risk is expected. Increased exercise, association with potential triggers such as horse hair/dander and increased exercise. Power Breathing is an asthma program specifically designed and pretested with the teen population. Knowledge, resilience and effectiveness in asthma self-care were measured before and after camp. All campers took home peak flow diaries with camp entries as well as spacers and peak flow meters.[3] What suggestions would you have for improvement of this program?

11. A British study of leaflets given before cataract surgery found that none stated that cataracts are normally harmless if left untreated or that there was a risk of losing an eye. Average readability was grade 10 with a range of 7 to 12. The leaflets' most common fault was an emphasis on benefits coupled with little attention to risks and side effects.[2] Are these serious faults?

12. A study of one end-stage renal disease (ESRD) network showed that the majority of patients were not presented with chronic peritoneal dialysis, home hemodialysis or renal transplantation as options. In the United States, more than 90% of patients undergo in-center maintenance hemodialysis.[9] Although comprehensive patient education programs are associated with a substantially higher selection of home dialysis and costs for providing it are consistently lower, pre-ESRD education

is not reimbursable. Why might patient education be less available to persons with ESRD than to persons with other chronic diseases?

13. Eighty percent of patients with congestive heart failure have memory deficits or other cognitive dysfunctions, at least in part the result of altered oxygen and nutrient supply to the brain because of decreased cardiac output. In a study of provision of care to these patients through a nurse-managed outpatient clinic or through conventional primary care, the questionnaire in Box 3 was used. It has been assessed by experts for content validity.[7] What is your critique of this questionnaire?

14. Capron[4] notes that, because "brain dead" patients show such traditional signs of life as warm, moist skin, a pulse, and breathing, it is not surprising that many people seem to think "brain death" is a separate type of death that occurs before "real" death. This confusion is reinforced when hospital personnel state that "life support" is being removed from such patients. Is it any wonder that families are confused?

ADDITIONAL CASE

1. Patients with cystic fibrosis have chronic infection of the airways and typical therapies include aerosolized medications. There is recent evidence that home nebulizers become contaminated by bacteria, causing concern that nebulizers may be a source of bacterial infection in the lower airways, aided by the excessive airway secretions these patients experience. Regular cleaning and drying and replacement of nebulizers can reduce bacterial contamination.

Although the Centers for Disease Control and Prevention suggest soaking the nebulizer in a mixture of one part bleach to 50 parts water for 3 minutes, 70% isopropyl alcohol for 5 minutes or 3% hydrogen peroxide for 30 minutes, the most widely used method (typically recommended by manufacturers in the nebulizer package insert) is soaking

Box 3	*The Heart Failure Knowledge Questionnaire*

A.1. Disease-specific Questions:

1. Do you know what congestive heart failure means?
2. Do you know who is at risk for congestive heart failure?
3. Do you know if patients with congestive heart failure should be vaccinated for influenza?
4. Should patients having congestive heart failure rest when feeling tired?

A.2. Questions and Statements about Self-care

5. Do you know if losing weight when overweight affects heart failure?
6. Why is quitting smoking positive for those with congestive heart failure?
7. Is there any simple method to verify signs of worsening heart failure?
8. Are you allowed to drink liquids as much as you want if you have congestive heart failure?
9. What are the most common symptoms of congestive heart failure?
10. What should a person with congestive heart failure do when having trouble with swelling legs?
11. What are considered fluids?
12. Why should you avoid sodium if you have congestive heart failure?
13. Should you avoid people with infections?
14. If you increase in weight more than two kilos and have signs of worsening heart failure, what should you do?
15. What kind of exercise is best when suffering from congestive heart failure?
16. What should you do if you have a fever?
17. Does alcohol decrease the working capacity of the heart?
18. Is it important to take diuretics at the same time every day?
19. If you have to take analgesics, which should you take?

From Karlsson and others: A nurse-based management program in heart failure patients affects females and persons with cognitive dysfunction most, *Patient Educ Couns* 58:146-153, 2005, used with permission.

in a solution of vinegar and water. A survey of patients in your hospital system shows that 15% use a disinfectant method at least once a week. A survey of respiratory therapists finds that they commonly recommend tap water or soap and water; only 41% of the respiratory therapists taught patients to use a disinfectant.[8] You're not certain if these practices are causing infections in the patients. What do you do?

SUGGESTED ANSWERS TO STUDY QUESTIONS

1. You first need to consider who loses money if the tests have to be redone because payment does constitute a reinforcer. Are patients disgusted with having to come back several times? Are other services in the hospital affected? It is likely that a good patient education program could improve bowel preparation, probably with increasing increments of improvements as the program and its delivery are refined.

2. This finding may say that no matter how much patients perform self-care behaviors as taught, their diabetes is not under control, which may mean that their medical treatments do not work very well. Under these circumstances, learning and doing self-care will not be reinforced because the patient continues to get worse. This finding may also reflect faulty self-reports on the patient's part.

3. Patient education can be designed to develop feelings of control by placing the patient in a major decision-making role in choice of treatment and by concentrating on development of self-efficacy for these behaviors.

4. Answers will vary.

5. (1) c, (2) b, (3) a, (4) b, (5) a, (6) c, (7) T, (8) T

6. a. Constructivist.
   b. That it will last because it has been constructed to make it meaningful to that individual.
   c. Listen to it, acknowledge it, and use it unless it is dangerous.

7. (1) Assessment allowing teaching targeted to each patient's needs and (2) teaching over a period of time, providing small doses of instruction over a number of months that could be incorporated into patients' daily self-care.

8. The findings should not be surprising because those with low numeracy could not easily understand how the changed instructions modified the dose. Patient education does not usually take on the instructional task of increasing numeracy (or literacy). Probably the only way to increase accuracy is to provide different dosages in standardized pill form and direct the patient which pill to take. It is doubtful that such patients can self-manage their regimens.

9. The hospital is not the best place to monitor the glycemic control of patients with diabetes because it is an unnatural environment in which diet is planned and activity is low.[12] Those with early discharge and continued nurse contact learned glycemic control in the environment in which they would manage it henceforth and gained increased self-efficacy with the supervision that ensured their success.

10. The objectives are not written to describe learner outcomes, which makes it difficult to determine whether participants learned or whether the camp was worth the investment. Learning occurs in an age-appropriate action environment. Participants are provided with equipment, use it, and interpret the results with learning help and in the company of peers—very important at this stage of development. The standard pretested program has been tested for effectiveness in this population. The before-and-after study design would be weak as a research study but acceptable for program evaluation.

11. They certainly are serious faults because the implicit purpose of the leaflets is to provide information toward informed consent for cataract surgery. Before consenting to treatment, patients have a right to know prognosis; treatment options including no treatment, risks and benefits, and costs to the patient.

12. Although diabetes education may be more available than is ESRD education, education for many chronic diseases is much less available that would seem warranted to accommodate patients' preferences, optimize quality of life, and control costs. Patient education has not historically been considered a medical intervention and certainly not a reimbursable one. Payment systems frequently reflect custom and physician preference, not patient well-being.

13. Questions 1 to 5 and to a lesser extent 7, 13, and 18 can be answered yes or no without testing the patient's knowledge. The reading level should be checked—do patients in your population understand "fluids," "sodium," "diuretics," "analgesics"? Question 14 assumes patient knowledge of "signs of worsening heart failure." This questionnaire does not test at higher levels of the cognitive domain such as integration and evaluation of knowledge, the very skills required to self-manage heart failure.

14. The answer is obvious.

SUGGESTED ANSWER TO CASE

1. Collecting systematic information on patients and respiratory therapists in your system is an important first step. How many of these patients have infections? The new standard issued by the Centers for Disease Control and Prevention (an authoritative government agency) must have been established on the basis of strong evidence, and if you don't ensure your institution is following it, you will not be meeting standards of care. These reliable, proven methods should be used both in the hospital and at home through a readily available and consistently distributed written, standard cleaning and replacement guide.[8] You will need to do follow-up audits to ensure compliance with this new standard and be able to take corrective action if it is not used.

REFERENCES

1. Barry MJ and others: Patient reactions to a program designed to facilitate patient participation in treatment decisions for benign prostatic hyperplasia, *Med Care* 33:771-782, 1995.

2. Brown H, Ramchandani M, Gillow JT, Tsaloumas MD: Are patient information leaflets contributing to informed consent for cataract surgery? *J Med Ethics* 30:218-220, 2004.

3. Buckner EB and others: Knowledge, resilience, and effectiveness of education in a young teen asthma camp, *Pediatr Nurs* 31:201-208, 2005.

4. Capron AM: Brain death—well settled yet still unresolved, *N Engl J Med* 344:1244-1246, 2001.

5. Estrada CA and others: Literacy and numeracy skills and anticoagulation control, *Am J Med Sci* 328:88-93, 2004.

6. Glasgow RE and others: Behavioral research on diabetes at the Oregon Research Institute, *Ann Behav Med* 17:32-40, 1995.

7. Karlsson MR and others: A nurse-based management program in heart failure patients affects females and persons with cognitive dysfunction most, *Patient Educ Couns* 58:146-153, 2005.

8. Lester MK and others: Nebulizer use and maintenance by cystic fibrosis patients: A survey study, *Respir Care* 49:1504-1508, 2004.

9. Mehrotra R and others: Patient education and access of ESRD patients to renal replacement therapies beyond in-center hemodialysis, *Kidney Int* 68:378-390, 2005.

10. Moser DK, Dracup K: Psychosocial recovery from a cardiac event: The influence of perceived control, *Heart Lung* 24:273-280, 1995.

11. Piette JD and others: Do automated calls with nurse follow-up improve self-care and glycemic control among vulnerable patients with diabetes? *Am J Med* 108:20-27, 2000.

12. Wong FKY, Mok MPH, Chan T, Tsang MW: Nurse follow-up of patients with diabetes: Randomized controlled trial, *J Adv Nurs* 50:391-402, 2005.

Index